Accident & Emergency Medicine
Data and Drug Guide

FRANCIS MORRIS MRCP FRCS
Consultant in Accident & Emergency Medicine,
Northern General Hospital, Sheffield

NIGEL KIDNER BSc MB ChB FRCS(Ed)
Senior Registrar in Accident & Emergency Medicine,
Northern General Hospital, Sheffield

CONOR KELLY MB ChB BAO FRCS
Senior Registrar in Accident & Emergency Medicine,
Royal Hospital, Wolverhampton

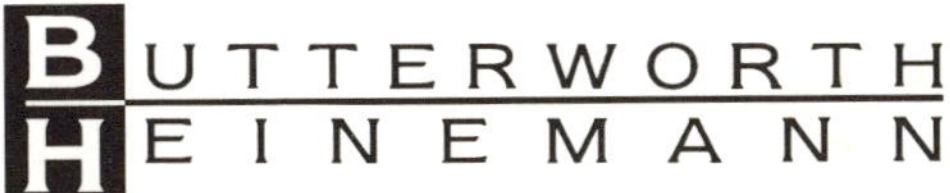

Butterworth-Heinemann Ltd
Linacre House, Jordan Hill, Oxford OX2 8DP

A member of the Reed Elsevier plc group

OXFORD LONDON BOSTON
MUNICH NEW DELHI SINGAPORE SYDNEY
TOKYO TORONTO WELLINGTON

First published 1995

British Library Cataloguing in Publication Data
A catalogue record for this book is available from the British Library.

ISBN 0 7506 2035 8

Library of Congress Cataloguing in Publication Data
A catalogue record for this book is available from the Library of Congress.

Printed in Great Britain by The University Press, Cambridge

Contents

Preface

Patients presenting to an Accident & Emergency Department are of all ages and present with a wide range of conditions. Many will require immediate assessment and management.

The sum total of clinical guidelines, normal values and drug data required to treat these patients is vast and overwhelming. It cannot be expected of the overstretched doctor to retain and recall all this information from memory. We have therefore compiled this book to provide a convenient and easily accessible source of vital information which will be of use to doctors, nurses and students working in accident & emergency medicine.

We have included current nationally agreed guidelines, drug data and other information of use in the A & E Department, concentrating on that which will be required in the emergency situation. Space and practicality, however, do not allow an exhaustive collection of data.

N.L.K.
C.K.
F.P.M.

Acknowledgements

We thank Mr J. Wardrope and Mr C. Chikhani for their comments, and Mrs Cynthia Hulbert for typing the manuscript. We also wish to acknowledge the following sources of data.

British Medical Journal Tavistock Square, London	Guidelines for the management of asthma *Br. Med. J.*, 1993; 306: 776–82
	Guidelines for the management of spontaneous pneumothorax *Br. Med. J.*, 1993; **307**: 114–16
	ABC of poisoning – non-poisons Henry, J. and Wiseman, H., *Br. Med. J.*, 1984; **289**: 240–1
	Peak Flow Normogram Gregg, I. and Nunn, A.J., *Br. Med. J.*, 1989; **298**: 1068–70
Resuscitation Elsevier Science Ireland Ltd	Adult cardiac arrest algorithms
Advanced Life Support Group, Manchester	Adult arrhythmia algorithms; paediatric arrhythmia and cardiac arrest algorithms; paediatric status epilepticus algorithm
Peter Oakley Anaesthesia/Trauma, Stoke-on-Trent	Paediatric resuscitation chart
C.J. Morley Department of Paediatrics, Cambridge	Baby Check
Royal College of Surgeons of England, London	Guidelines on sedation *Ann. R. Coll. Surg. Engl.*, supplement 1993;
European Resuscitation Council (UK)	Guideline for bradycardia, broad complex tachycardia and narrow complex tachycardia algorithms

S. Godfrey	Peak expiratory flow in normal children (age 6-15 years). *Br. J. Dis. Chest*, **64**: 15–24
British Association for Accident & Emergency Medicine	Management of acute poisoning
National Poisons Information Service, London	Paracetamol overdose Paracetamol poisoning treatment graph

Abbreviations

AV	atrioventricular
BP	blood pressure
CCF	congestive cardiac failure
CPR	cardio-pulmonory resuscitation
CSM	Committee on Safety of Medicines
CVA	cerebrovascular accident
DM	diabetes mellitus
EMD	electromechanical dissociation
GI	gastrointestinal
HR	heart rate
INR	International Normalized Ratio
LFT	liver function tests
MI	myocardial infarction
PEF	peak expiratory flow
SVT	supraventricular tachycardia
VF	ventricular fibrillation
VT	ventricular tachycardia
WBC	white blood-cell count
i.m.	intramuscular
i.o.	intraosseous
i.v.	intravenous
p.r.	per rectum
q.d.s.	four times a day
s.c.	subcutaneous
t.d.s.	three times a day
S/E	side effects

Resuscitation Protocols and Guidelines

ADULT

Ventricular fibrillation (VF) or pulseless ventricular tachycardia (VT)

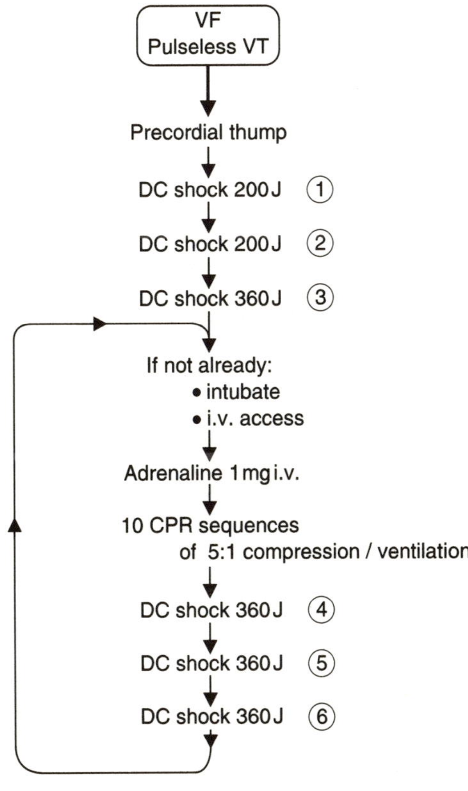

Notes: (i) The interval between shocks 3 and 4 should not be >2 min.
(ii) Adrenaline given during loop approx. every 2–3 min.
(iii) Continue loops for as long as defibrillation is indicated.
(iv) After 3 loops consider:
- an alkalizing agent
- an antiarrhythmic agent

ADULT

Asystole

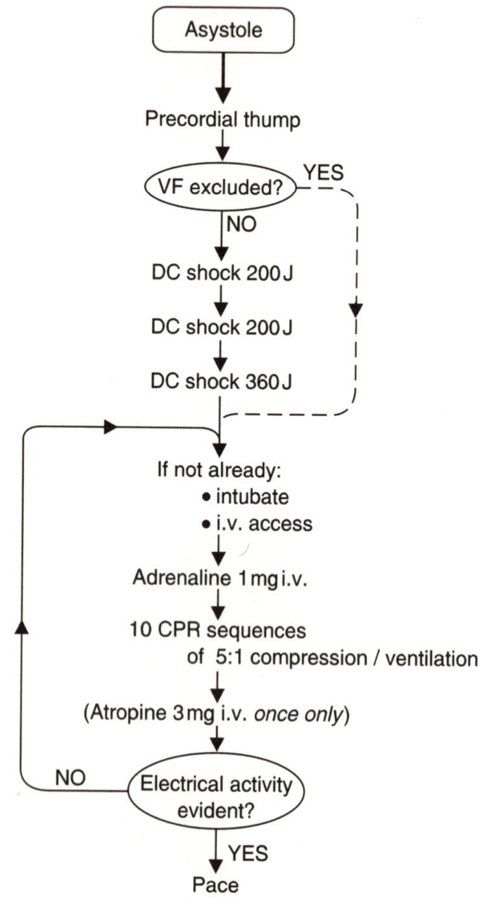

Note: If no response after 3 cycles consider high dose adrenaline: 5mg i.v.

ADULT

Electromechanical dissociation (EMD)

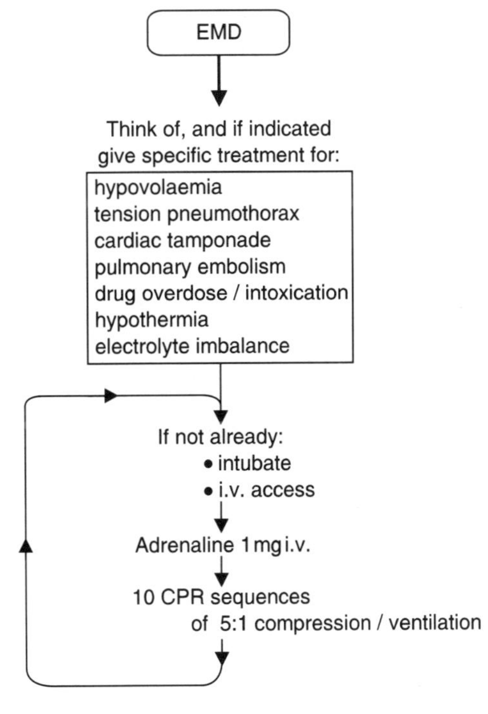

CONSIDER
- Pressor agents
- Calcium
- Alkalizing agents
- Adrenaline 5 mg i.v.

ADULT

Supraventricular tachycardia

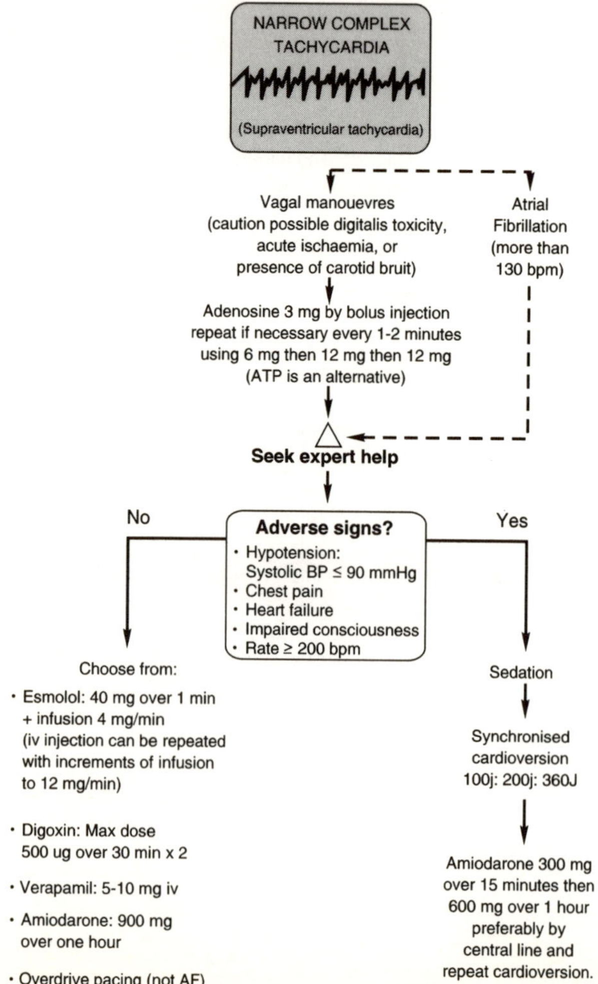

ADULT

Wide complex tachycardias

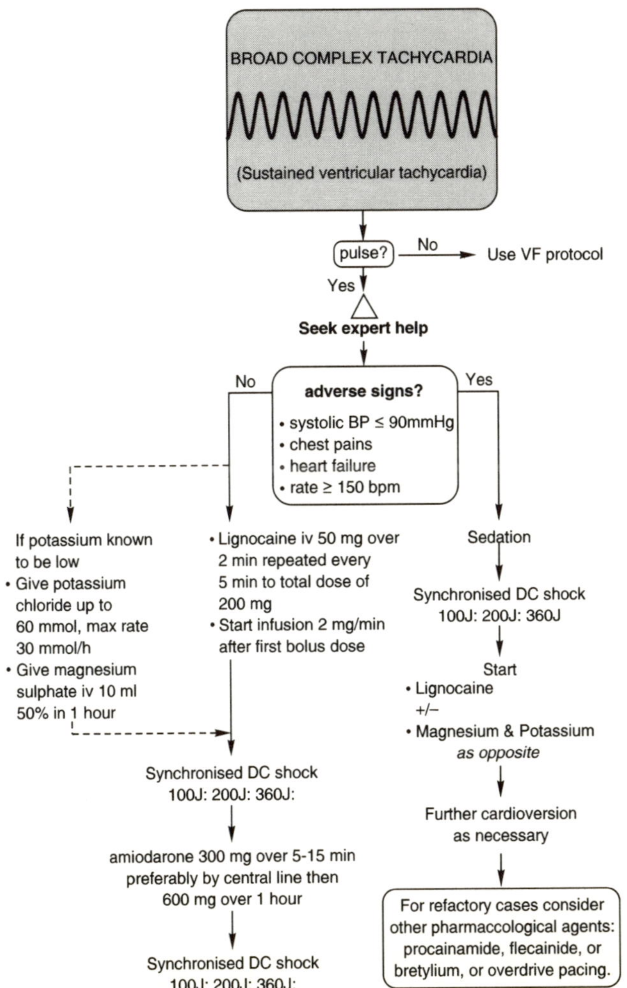

ADULT

Bradycardias

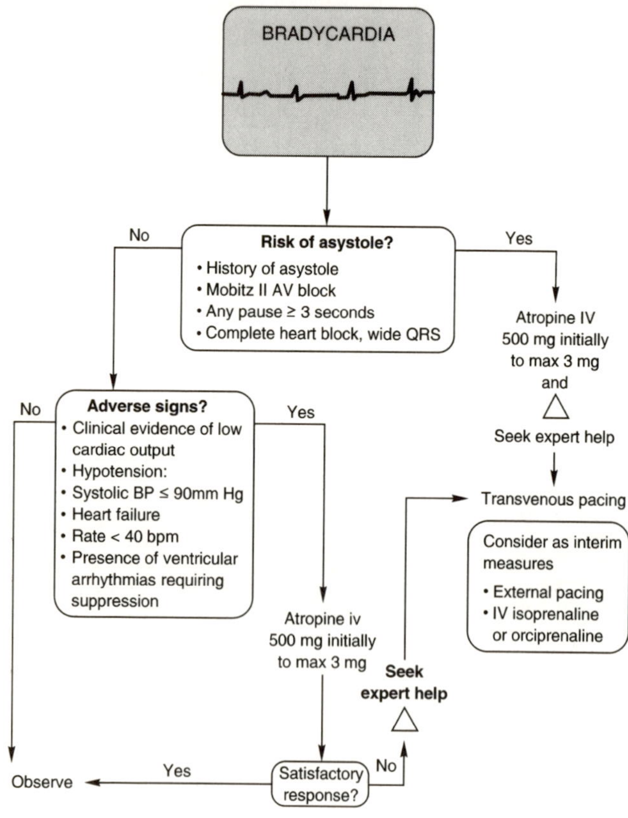

PAEDIATRIC

Ventricular fibrillation

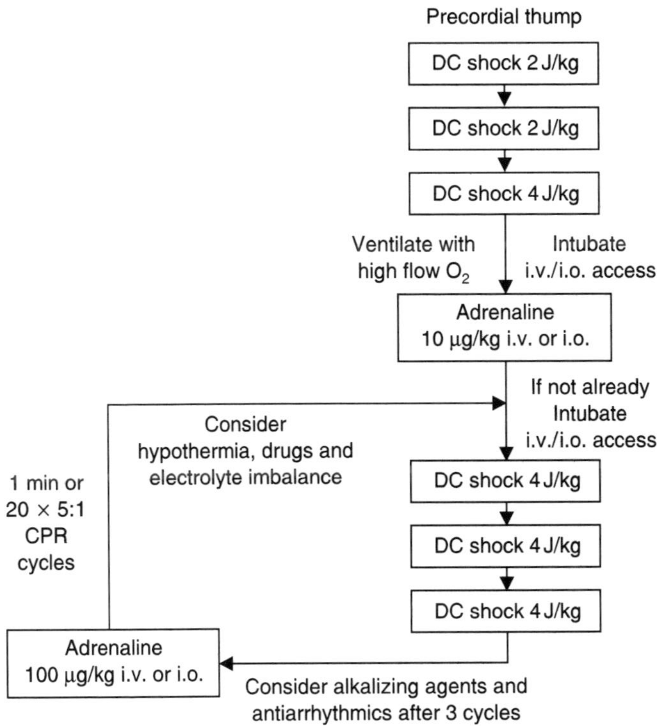

PAEDIATRIC

Asystole

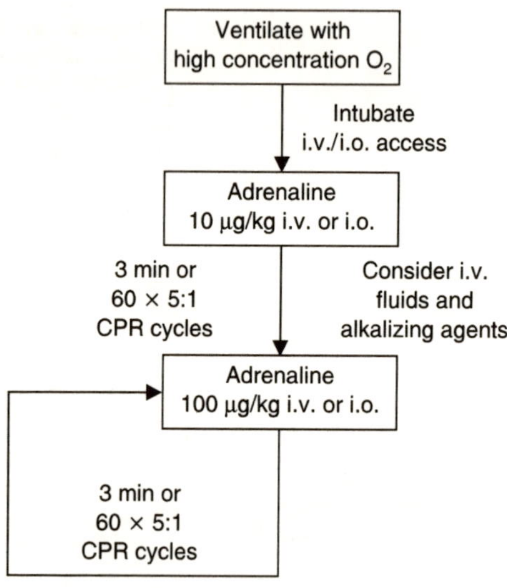

PAEDIATRIC

Electromechanical dissociation (EMD)

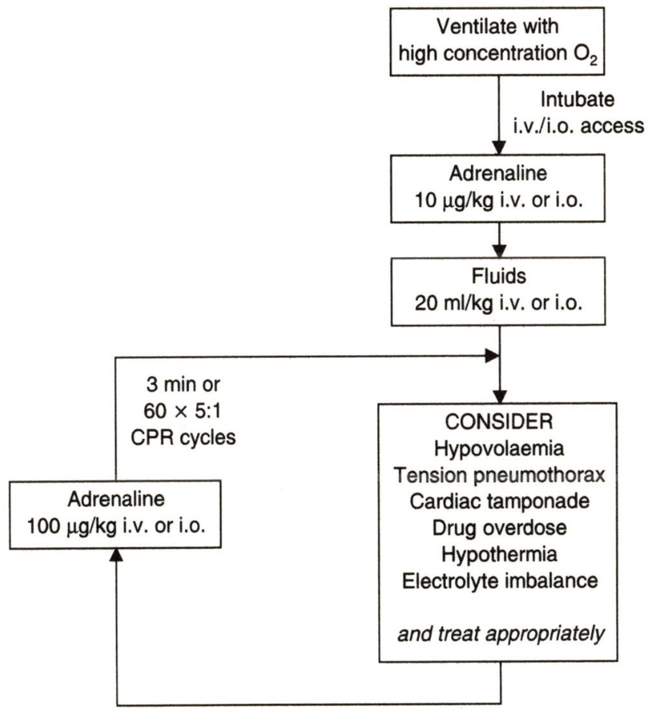

PAEDIATRIC

Supraventricular tachycardia

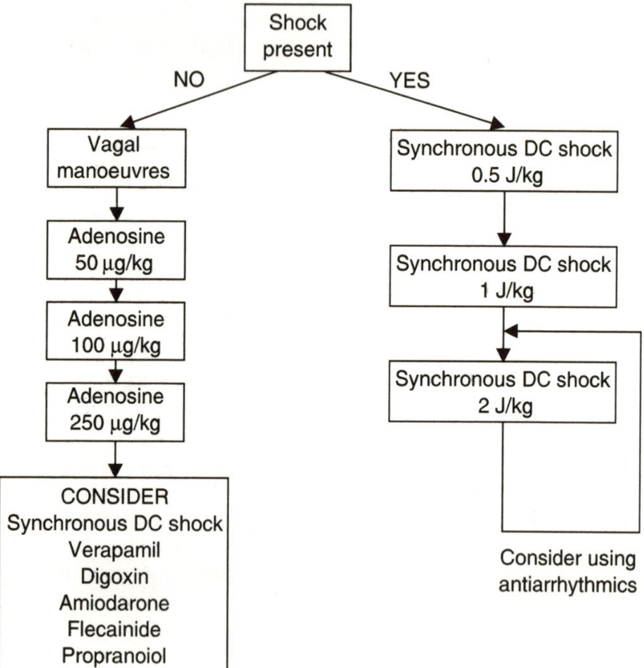

PAEDIATRIC

Ventricular tachycardia

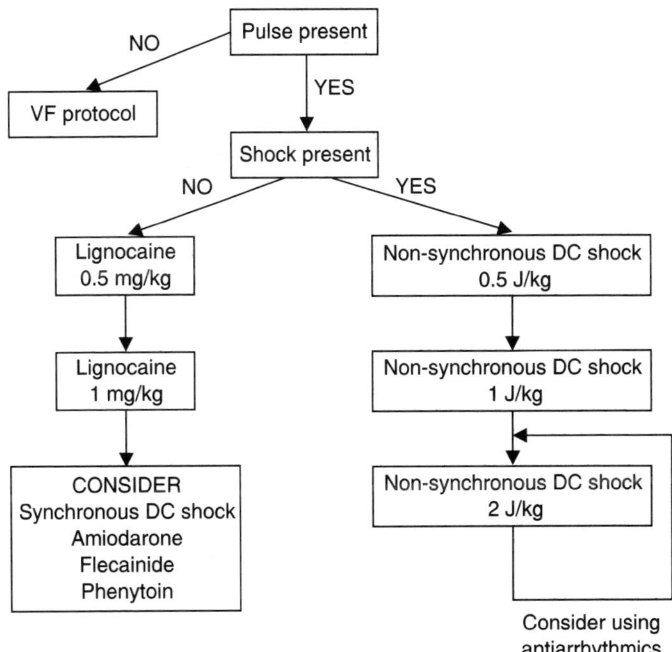

PAEDIATRIC

Bradycardias

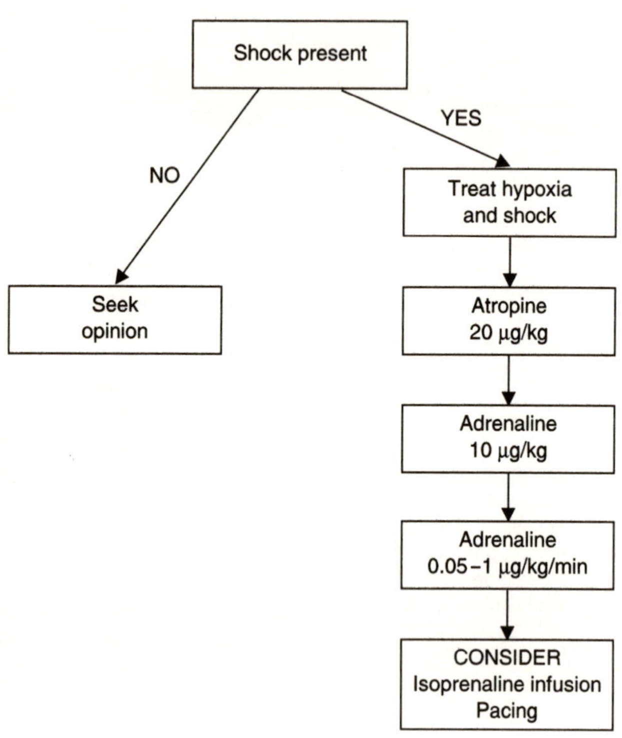

Paediatric resuscitation chart

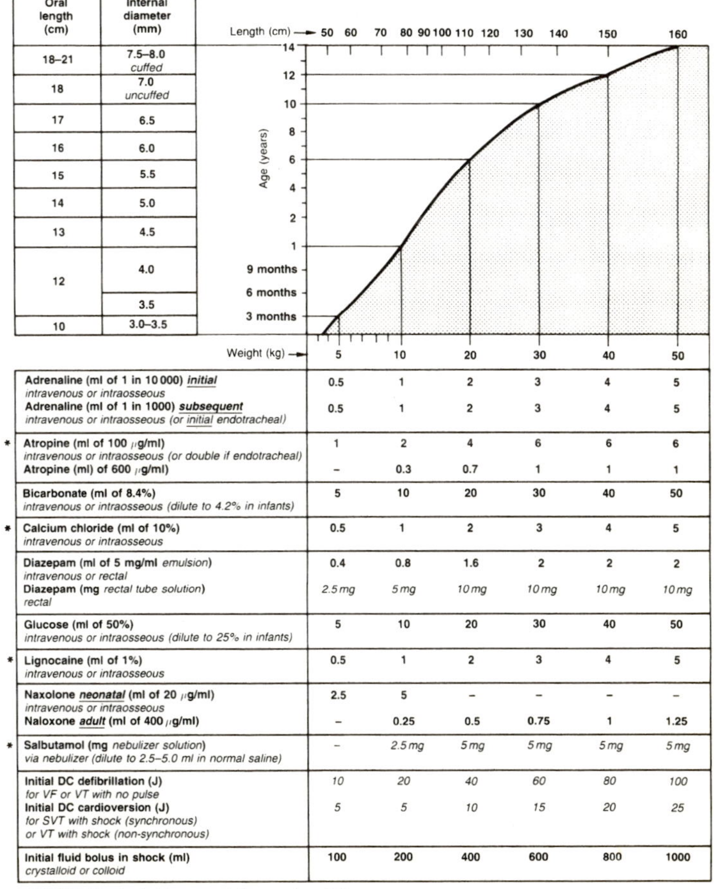

Endotracheal tube

Oral length (cm)	Internal diameter (mm)
18–21	7.5–8.0 *cuffed*
18	7.0 *uncuffed*
17	6.5
16	6.0
15	5.5
14	5.0
13	4.5
12	4.0
	3.5
10	3.0–3.5

Weight (kg)	5	10	20	30	40	50
Adrenaline (ml of 1 in 10 000) *initial* *intravenous or intraosseous*	0.5	1	2	3	4	5
Adrenaline (ml of 1 in 1000) *subsequent* *intravenous or intraosseous (or initial endotracheal)*	0.5	1	2	3	4	5
* **Atropine (ml of 100 μg/ml)** *intravenous or intraosseous (or double if endotracheal)*	1	2	4	6	6	6
Atropine (ml) of 600 μg/ml)	–	0.3	0.7	1	1	1
Bicarbonate (ml of 8.4%) *intravenous or intraosseous (dilute to 4.2% in infants)*	5	10	20	30	40	50
* **Calcium chloride (ml of 10%)** *intravenous or intraosseous*	0.5	1	2	3	4	5
Diazepam (ml of 5 mg/ml *emulsion*) *intravenous or rectal*	0.4	0.8	1.6	2	2	2
Diazepam (mg *rectal tube solution*) *rectal*	*2.5 mg*	*5 mg*	*10 mg*	*10 mg*	*10 mg*	*10 mg*
Glucose (ml of 50%) *intravenous or intraosseous (dilute to 25% in infants)*	5	10	20	30	40	50
* **Lignocaine (ml of 1%)** *intravenous or intraosseous*	0.5	1	2	3	4	5
Naxolone *neonatal* (ml of 20 μg/ml) *intravenous or intraosseous*	2.5	5	–	–	–	–
Naloxone *adult* (ml of 400 μg/ml)	–	0.25	0.5	0.75	1	1.25
* **Salbutamol (mg** *nebulizer solution*) *via nebulizer (dilute to 2.5–5.0 ml in normal saline)*	–	*2.5 mg*	*5 mg*	*5 mg*	*5 mg*	*5 mg*
Initial DC defibrillation (J) *for VF or VT with no pulse*	*10*	*20*	*40*	*60*	*80*	*100*
Initial DC cardioversion (J) *for SVT with shock (synchronous)* *or VT with shock (non-synchronous)*	*5*	*5*	*10*	*15*	*20*	*25*
Initial fluid bolus in shock (ml) *crystalloid or colloid*	100	200	400	600	800	1000

* ***CAUTION!*** *Non-standard drug concentrations may be available:*
Use ***Atropine*** *100 μg/ml or prepare by diluting 1 mg to 10 ml or 600 μg to 6 ml in normal saline.*
Note that 1 ml of ***calcium chloride*** *10% is equivalent to 3 ml of* ***calcium gluconate*** *10%.*
Use ***Lignocaine*** *(without adrenaline) 1% or give twice the volume of 0.5%. Give half the volume of 2% or dilute appropriately.*
Salbutamol may also be given by slow intravenous injection (5 μg/kg), but beware of the different concentrations available (eg 50 and 500 μg/ml).

Paediatric Data

Vital signs

Blood pressure (mmHg) = 80 + (age × 2)

	Age (yr)		
	< 1	*2–5*	*5–12*
Heart rate	120–140	100–120	80–100
Blood pressure	70–90	80–90	90–110
Respiratory rate	30–40	20–30	15–20

Body weight (kg) = (age + 4) × 2

Apgar score

Measure at 1 minute and 5 minutes

Sign	**0**	**1**	**2**
Heart rate	Nil	<100	>100
Respiratory effort	Nil	Slow, irregular	Good, crying
Muscle tone	Limp	Some flexion limbs	Active motion
Reflex irritability	No response	Grimace	Cry, cough
Colour	Blue	Body Extremities blue	Completely pink

Apgar score is a numerical assessment of baby's condition at birth: it is not particularly useful in predicting which babies require resuscitation as this is based on respiration and pulse.

Initial resuscitation of a newborn

Category	Initial findings	Action
Healthy	Pink HR >100 Good respiratory effort	Dry Keep warm Give to mother
Primary apnoea	Blue HR >80 Apnoeic or gasping	Gentle suction O_2 by mask ?Bag/mask ventilation
Terminal apnoea	White Heart rate <80 Apnoeic	Gentle suction Bag/mask ventilation ?Intubation
Fresh stillbirth	White Asystolic Apnoeic	Intubation Cardiac compression ?Drugs

Endotracheal tubes

Tracheal tube internal diameter (mm)
(Age/4) + 4.5
Tracheal tube length (cm)
Oral: Age/2 + 12
Nasal: Age/2 + 15

Baby Check

The Baby Check has been designed for use by parents but it acts as a useful '*aide-mémoire*' for junior doctors with little paediatric experience.

INSTRUCTIONS

- **Baby Check** contains 19 simple checks.
- Each check tests for a different symptom or sign of illness.
- Each check has a score. As you go through the checks, you add up the scores.
- All checks must be scored for the total score to assess accurately the baby's illness.
- The interpretation of the total score is shown on p. 25.
- The higher the score the sicker the baby is likely to be.
- Score each check according to the exact wording of the question.
- Only score it a check is obviously present.
- **Baby Check** is not a substitute for clinical judgement or common sense.
- **Baby Check** assesses symptoms and signs of generalized illness. Some conditions, such as injury, a convulsion or abscess, where the baby is not systemically ill, may get a low score but still need medical assessment or treatment.
- The baby can be re-scored at any time to assess changes in the severity of the illness.
- The score indicates the severity of an illness at the time it is done. It is not prognostic.
- **Baby Check** is not designed to assess babies with chronic conditions.

References

1. Morley, C.J. *et al.* (1990) *Recent Advances in Paediatrics*, Churchill Livingstone, ch. 9
2. Morley, C.J., Thornton, A.J. *et al.* (1991) *Archives of Disease in Childhood*, **66**: 100–120

THE CHECKS

Have these symptoms been present in the last 24 hours?

		SCORE
1.	Has the baby vomited at least half the feed after each of the last three feeds?	**4**
2.	Has the baby had any bile-stained (green) vomiting?	**13**
3.	Has the baby taken less **fluids** than usual in the last 24 hours? If so score for the total amount of fluids taken as follows:	
	• Taken slightly less than usual (more than $\frac{2}{3}$ normal)	**3**
	• Taken about half usual amount $\frac{1}{3}-\frac{2}{3}$ normal)	**4**
	• Taken very little (less than $\frac{1}{3}$ normal)	**9**
	★ *Breast feeding mothers should estimate the amount taken.*	
	★ *Fluids that have been vomited should still be scored.*	
4.	Has the baby passed less urine than usual?	**3**
5.	Has there been any frank blood (not streaks) mixed with the baby's stools?	**11**
6.	Has the baby been *drowsy* (less alert than usual) *when awake*? If so, score as follows:	
	• Occasionally drowsy (but *usually* alert)	**3**
	• Drowsy most of the time (*occasionally* alert)	**5**
	★ *Do not score irritability or increased sleeping.*	
7.	Has the baby had an unusual cry (sounds unusual to mother)?	**2**

Now examine the baby awake

8.	Is the baby more floppy than you would expect?	**4**

		SCORE
9.	Talk to the baby. Is the baby watching you less than you expect?	**4**
10.	Is the baby wheezing (not snuffles or upper respiratory noises on expiration)?	**3**
11.	Is the baby responding less than you would expect to what is going on around?	**5**

Now examine the baby **naked** *for the following checks*

12.	Is there any indrawing (recession) of the lower ribs, sternum or upper abdomen? If so, score as follows:	
	• just visible with each breath?	**4**
	• obvious and deep indrawing with each breath?	**15**
13.	Is the baby abnormally pale or has the baby looked very pale in the last 24 hours?	**3**
14.	Does the baby have blue fingernails or toenails?	**3**
15.	Squeeze the big toe to make it white. Release and observe colour for 3 seconds. Score if the toe is not pink within 3 seconds, or if it was completely white to start with.	**3**
16.	Has the baby got an inguinal hernia?	**13**
17.	Has the baby an obvious generalized truncal rash or a sore and weeping rash covering an area greater than 5 × 5 cm?	**4**
18.	Is the baby's rectal temperature 38.3°C or more?	**4**
19.	Has the baby cried (more than just a grizzle) during this assessment?	**3**

Total score . . . .

The higher the score the sicker the baby. For interpretation of the scores ***see p. 25***

Interpretation of the scores

This table shows the chance of a baby being well or mildly ill, moderately ill or seriously ill at different scores. (The positive predictive value of the scores.)

Score	Well or mildly ill	Moderately ill	Seriously ill
0	99%	1%	0%
2	90%	9%	1%
4	85%	14%	2%
6	77%	21%	2%
8	66%	30%	4%
10	54%	41%	5%
12	41%	51%	8%
14	30%	58%	12%
16	20%	62%	18%
18	13%	62%	25%
20	8%	58%	34%
22	5%	50%	45%
24	3%	41%	56%
26	2%	32%	66%
28	1%	24%	75%
30	0%	17%	83%
32	0%	12%	88%
34	0%	8%	92%
36	0%	5%	95%
38	0%	3%	97%
40	0%	2%	98%
42	0%	1%	99%
48	0%	0%	100%

Example: A baby scoring 24 has a 3% chance of being well or mildly ill, a 41% chance of being moderately ill and a 56% chance of being seriously ill.

Score groups and advice used in the parent's booklet

The higher the score the sicker your baby is likely to be.

Score 0 to 7	Your baby is well or only a little unwell and is not likely to need medical attention now.
Score 8 to 12	Your baby is unwell, but not likely to be seriously ill at the moment. Contact your doctor, health visitor or midwife for advice. Watch your baby closely: if you think your baby is worse, do the score again.
Score 13 to 19	Your baby is ill and needs to be seen by a doctor. Contact your doctor **now** and arrange for your baby to be seen.
Score 20+	Your baby may be seriously ill and needs to be seen by a doctor straight away.

Copies for professionals or parents can be obtained from: Baby Check, PO Box 324, Wroxham, Norwich NR12 8EQ. Tel (01603) 784400.

Information can be obtained from Dr C. Morley, Dept of Paediatrics, Level 8, Addenbrooke's Hospital, Cambridge, CB2 2QQ.

Status epilepticus

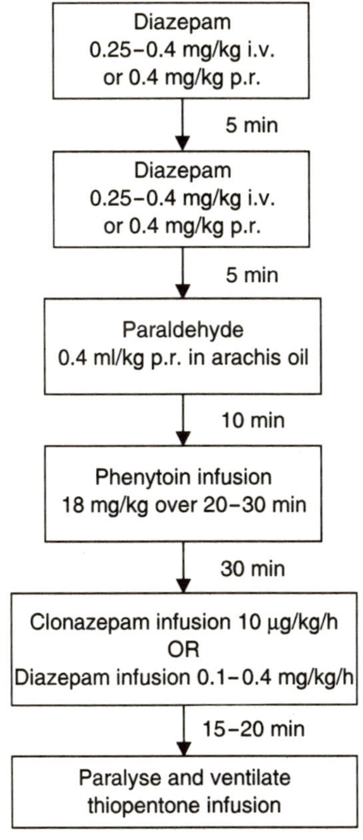

Immunization schedule (UK)

INFANT

Birth	BCG for babies in Asian and other immigrant families with high TB rates or those in contact with active respiratory TB
2 months	Polio and diphtheria/tetanus/pertussis (DPT) and haemophilus influenza B (HIB)
3 months	Polio and DPT and HIB
4 months	Polio and DPT and HIB
12–18 months	Combined measles/mumps/rubella (MMR) or measles (preferably 15 months)
12–48 months	HIB if not given before

PRE-SCHOOL

4–5 years	MMR if not previously given Polio and diphtheria/tetanus booster

SECONDARY SCHOOL

10–14 years	Heaf or Mantoux and, if negative, BCG
10–14 years	Rubella (girls only)

SCHOOL LEAVING

15–19 years	Polio and tetanus

Acute Medicine

Asthma

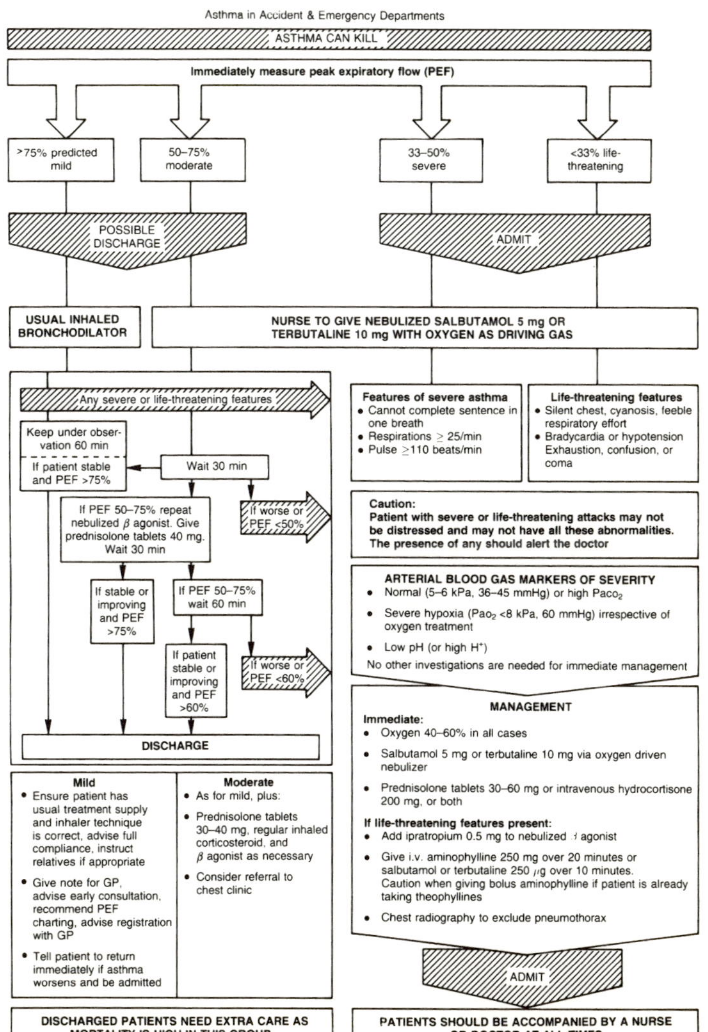

Asthma in Accident & Emergency Departments
ASTHMA CAN KILL
Immediately measure peak expiratory flow (PEF)
>75% predicted mild
50–75% moderate
33–50% severe
<33% life-threatening
POSSIBLE DISCHARGE
ADMIT
USUAL INHALED BRONCHODILATOR
NURSE TO GIVE NEBULIZED SALBUTAMOL 5 mg OR TERBUTALINE 10 mg WITH OXYGEN AS DRIVING GAS
Any severe or life-threatening features
Keep under observation 60 min
If patient stable and PEF >75%
Wait 30 min
If PEF 50–75% repeat nebulized β agonist. Give prednisolone tablets 40 mg. Wait 30 min
If worse or PEF <50%
If stable or improving and PEF >75%
If PEF 50–75% wait 60 min
If patient stable or improving and PEF >60%
If worse or PEF <60%
DISCHARGE
Features of severe asthma
• Cannot complete sentence in one breath
• Respirations ≥ 25/min
• Pulse ≥110 beats/min
Life-threatening features
• Silent chest, cyanosis, feeble respiratory effort
• Bradycardia or hypotension Exhaustion, confusion, or coma
Caution:
Patient with severe or life-threatening attacks may not be distressed and may not have all these abnormalities. The presence of any should alert the doctor
ARTERIAL BLOOD GAS MARKERS OF SEVERITY
• Normal (5–6 kPa, 36–45 mmHg) or high Paco2
• Severe hypoxia (Pao2 <8 kPa, 60 mmHg) irrespective of oxygen treatment
• Low pH (or high H+)
No other investigations are needed for immediate management
MANAGEMENT
Immediate:
• Oxygen 40–60% in all cases
• Salbutamol 5 mg or terbutaline 10 mg via oxygen driven nebulizer
• Prednisolone tablets 30–60 mg or intravenous hydrocortisone 200 mg, or both
If life-threatening features present:
• Add ipratropium 0.5 mg to nebulized β agonist
• Give i.v. aminophylline 250 mg over 20 minutes or salbutamol or terbutaline 250 μg over 10 minutes. Caution when giving bolus aminophylline if patient is already taking theophyllines
• Chest radiography to exclude pneumothorax
ADMIT
Mild
• Ensure patient has usual treatment supply and inhaler technique is correct, advise full compliance, instruct relatives if appropriate
• Give note for GP, advise early consultation, recommend PEF charting, advise registration with GP
• Tell patient to return immediately if asthma worsens and be admitted
Moderate
• As for mild, plus:
• Prednisolone tablets 30–40 mg, regular inhaled corticosteroid, and β agonist as necessary
• Consider referral to chest clinic
DISCHARGED PATIENTS NEED EXTRA CARE AS MORTALITY IS HIGH IN THIS GROUP
PATIENTS SHOULD BE ACCOMPANIED BY A NURSE OR DOCTOR AT ALL TIMES
This chart is appropriate for patients from puberty onwards

Peak expiratory flow in normal adults

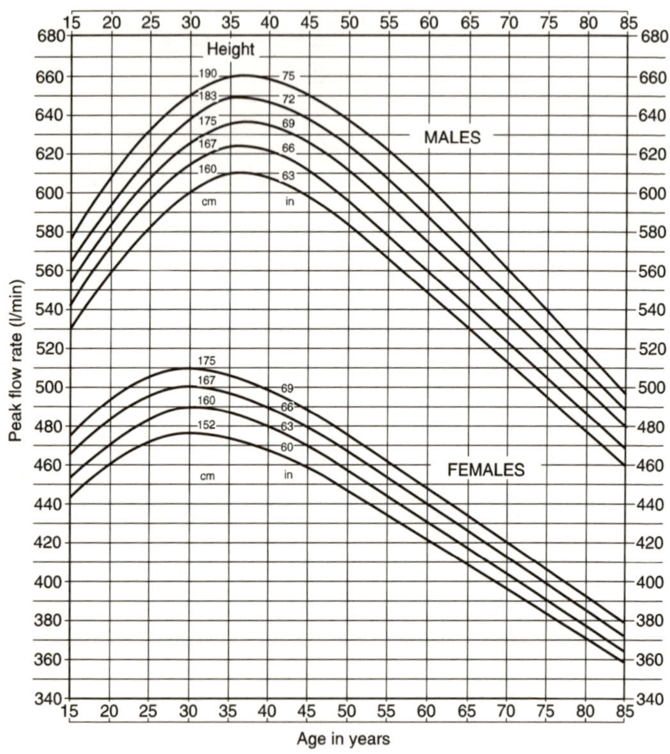

Peak expiratory flow in normal children (age 6–15 years)

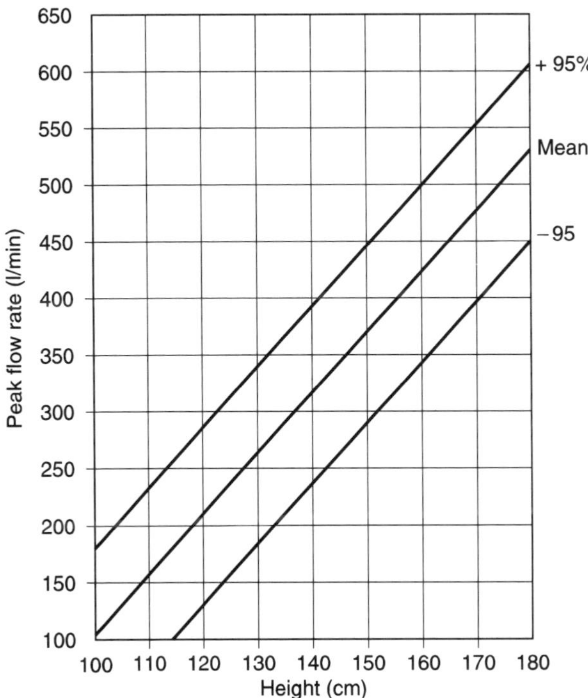

This nomogram results from tests carried out by Dr S. Godfrey and his colleagues on a sample of 382 normal boys and girls aged 5–18 years. Each child blew five times into a standard Wright Peak Flow Meter and the highest reading was accepted in each case. All measurements were completed within a 6-week period. The outer lines of the graph indicated that the results of 95% of the children fell within these boundaries. (Godfrey *et al.* (1970) *Br. J. Dis. Chest*, **64**: 15–24.)

Pneumothorax

Treatment of pneumothoraces depends upon the degree of collapse, the patient's symptoms and the presence of underlying chronic lung disease.

The following treatment guidelines are adapted from the British Thoracic Society Recommendations.

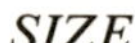

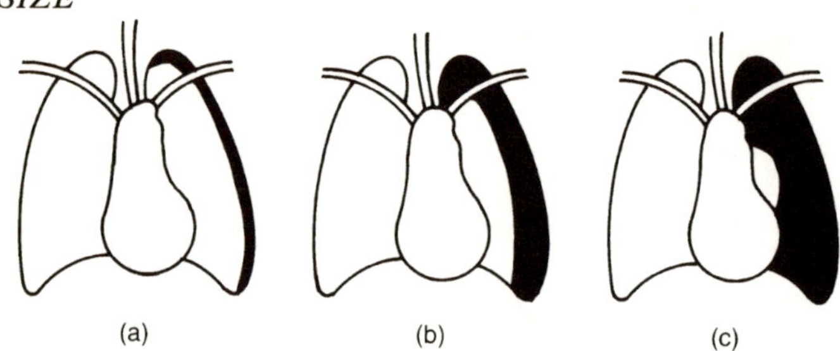

IF SIGNIFICANT DYSPNOEA OR UNDERLYING CHRONIC LUNG DISEASE:

Aspirate (a)	Drain (b)	Drain (c)

IF NO SIGNIFICANT DYSPNOEA:

Observe in hospital (a)	Aspirate (b)	Drain (c)

TENSION PNEUMOTHORAX: immediate decompression with a needle and syringe, followed by definitive intercostal drainage

TRAUMATIC PNEUMOTHORAX: drain all and admit to cardiothoracic surgical unit

Note: SIGNIFICANT DYSPNOEA: this means an obvious deterioration in usual exercise tolerance. Aspiration is necessary. If aspiration has been successful observe in hospital. If not insert a formal drain.

Management of acute poisoning

TREATMENT OF UNRESPONSIVE PATIENTS

A • Clear and secure the airway
Give high concentration (>40%) oxygen via mask and reservoir bag
Pulse oximeter

If the gag response is depressed insert a cuffed endotracheal tube
Get anaesthetic help

B • Assist ventilation if respiration is inadequate
Consider 0.8 mg naloxone i.v. and/or i.m. in patients with
A history of narcotic overdose
Depressed ventilation or conscious level
Pin-point pupils
The dose must be titrated against the clinical response
Repeated doses are almost always required
Consider infusion of naloxone

C • Insert an intravenous cannula. Attach the patient to an ECG monitor
Check blood glucose using reagent strips. If the reading is low give 50 ml 50% dextrose (children 1 ml/kg) (alternative Glucagon 1mg)
Send blood samples for
Laboratory measurement of plasma glucose and urea and electrolytes
Arterial blood gas determinations
Serum paracetamol and salicylate levels
Save serum

- Treat significant hypotension with a plasma expander
- Do not treat cardiac dysrhythmias provided the patient is maintaining an acceptable blood pressure
- Correct any metabolic acidosis which persists after hypoxia and hypercapnia have been abolished
- Treat recurrent or protracted fits with i.v. diazepam titrated against the response

- Hypothermic patients should be wrapped in a polythene sheet and nursed in a warm room
- Do not pronounce death until the victim has been rewarmed

Treatment of paracetamol poisoning

Treatment recommended following ingestion of more than 5 g by an adult and 150 mg/kg by a child

Some patients are more susceptible, e.g. those with induced liver enzymes, e.g. alcoholics and patients on anticonvulsants

< 4 HOURS POST INGESTION

- Empty stomach – gastric lavage (adult) – ipecacuanha (child)
- Activated charcoal – need ratio of 10:1 to paracetamol
- Blood level at 4 hours
- If TOXIC – oral methionine
  – i.v. N-acetylcysteine (if unconscious, vomiting or has just been given charcoal)

4–8 HOURS POST INGESTION

- Immediate measurement of plasma concentration
- If TOXIC treat as above (lavage, ipecacuanha or charcoal *unlikely to be of any use*)

8–10 HOURS POST INGESTION

- Oral methionine or i.v. N-acetylcysteine immediately without available level
- If level is NON TOXIC, *STOP ANTIDOTE*

10–24 HOURS POST INGESTION

- Give N-acetylcysteine immediately without available level
- If level NON TOXIC, *STOP ANTIDOTE*

24–36 HOURS POST INGESTION

- Give i.v. N-acetylcysteine if strong history of toxic ingestion
- Check levels, INR and LFTs
- If no clinical signs of hepatotoxicity, INR < 2, normal LFTs and non-detectable levels of paracetamol, *STOP ANTIDOTE*

> 36 HOURS POST INGESTION AND SIGNS OF HEPATOTOXICITY

- Discuss with nearest liver unit

INDICATIONS FOR REFERRAL

(A) INR >2.0 at 24 hours
INR >4.0 at 48 hours
INR >6.0 at 72 hours
(B) Elevated creatinine
(C) Evidence of encephalopathy
(D) Hypotension following volume replacement
(E) Metabolic acidosis with pH <7.3

Paracetamol poisoning treatment graph

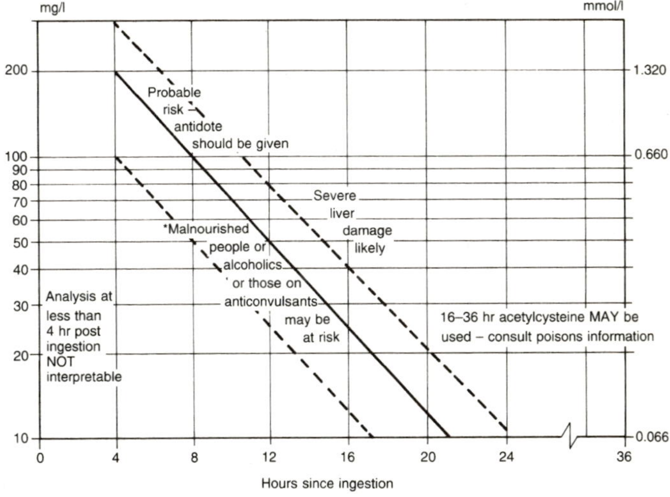

*Guide only, not based on published data

Non-poisons

DRUGS

- Antibiotics
- Vitamins without iron
- Simple antacids
- Oral contraceptives (possible withdrawal bleed in girls over 4)
- Homeopathic preparations
- Skin creams
  zinc oxide
  titanium oxide
  calamine lotion
  petroleum jelly
  Vaseline
  lanolin
  silicone

PLANTS

- *Berries*
  berberis spp.
  Chinese lantern
  cotoneaster spp.
  hawthorn
  mahonia spp.
  mountain ash/rowan
  pyracantha spp.
  Skimmia japonica

- *Flowers* (most are non-toxic), e.g.
  antirhinum
  daffodil
  bluebell
  daisy
  dandelion
  fuschia
  geranium

orchid
rose
violet
NB: **BULBS ARE TOXIC**

- *Leaves*
  African violet
  amalia
  begonia
  Busy Lizzie
  cacti (household)
  cheese plant
  cyclamen
  draconia
  rubber plant
  spider plant
  umbrella plant
  yucca

HOUSEHOLD PRODUCTS

- Chalk
- Crayons
- Felt tip pens
- Indelible markers
- Paints
  children's water colours
  colour blocks
  powder colours
  emulsion paint
  NB: **Artists' paint may contain toxic pigments**

SOAPS AND DETERGENTS

- Bar soaps
- Bubble bath
- Carpet cleaner
- Dishwashing liquid (**NOT POWDER – HIGHLY ALKALINE**)

- Dishwashing rinse aid
- Fabric soakers
- Fabric softeners
- Fabric washing powders and flakes
- Fabric rinse conditioner
- Shaving foam and soaps
- Scouring powders and scourers
- General purpose cleaning liquid and powder

COSMETICS

- Bath oil
- Bath foam
- Cleansing cream
- Cream for hands and body
- Dental disclosing tablets
- Hair conditioner, gel
- Lipstick
- Make-up for face and eyes
- Oils for skin and hair
- Suntan preparations
- Toothpaste
- Talc (NB: **MAY CAUSE ACUTE BRONCHITIS IF INHALED**)

NB: Nail varnish and nail varnish remover contain toxic solvents
Most perfumes contain alcohol
Hair dyes containing permanent dyes may contain ammonia

BUT: Toxic amounts are rarely absorbed

MISCELLANEOUS

- Candles (beeswax or paraffin)
- Lubricants, mineral oil
- Modelling clay
- Plasticine
- Blu-tac

- Putty
- Newspaper
- Silica gel
- Sweetening agents, e.g. saccharine
- Starch
- Water-based pastes, gums and adhesives (as opposed to hydrocarbon solvents)

Poison information services

Belfast	01232 240503
Birmingham	0121 5543801
Cardiff	01222 709901
Edinburgh	0131 2292477
Leeds	01132 430715
London	0171 6359191
	0171 9555095
Newcastle	0191 2325131
Dublin	01 8379964/6 (from RoI)

Contraindications to thrombolysis

Absolute	*Relative*
1. Active GI bleeding or active internal bleeding (including menstruation)	1. Traumatic CPR
2. Aortic dissection	2. Major surgery 10/7
3. Neurosurgery/head injury <2/12	3. Systolic BP >200 if not controllable Diastolic BP >130
4. CVA <2/12	4. Previous GI bleeding <6/12
5. Intracranial neoplasm/aneurysm	5. Abdominal aneurysm
6. Bleeding diathesis or thrombocytopenia or other evidence of haemostasis	6. Subclavian puncture
	7. Serious trauma Recent delivery (10/7)
	8. Ulcerative colitis
	9. Proliferative DM retinopathy

Notifiable diseases (UK)

CENTRAL NERVOUS SYSTEM

Acute meningitis (*E, W, NI*)
Polio
Acute encephalitis (*E, W*)
Encephalitis lethargica (*S*)
Meningococcal infection
Tetanus
Rabies

GASTROINTESTINAL

Cholera
Dysentery
Typhus
Paratyphoid
Food poisoning
Gastroenteritis (*under 2 yr NI*)
Infectious hepatitis (A)
Hepatitis (B)
Leptospirosis (*E, W*)

GENERAL

Scarlet fever
Measles
Rubella
Chicken pox (*S, NI*)
Mumps
Relapsing fever

IMPORTED

Malaria (*E, W, S*)
Typhus

Smallpox
Plague
Yellow fever (*E, W, NI*)
Leprosy (*E, W, S*)

SKIN AND MUCOUS MEMBRANES

Erysipelas (*S*)
Leprosy (*E, W, S*)
Anthrax
Ophthalmia neonatorum (*E, W, S*)

RESPIRATORY SYSTEM

Diphtheria
Pneumonia
Tuberculosis (respiratory and non-respiratory)
Whooping cough
Legionnaire's disease

GENITO-URINARY

Puerperal fever or pyrexia
Sexually transmitted diseases:
- Gonorrhoea
- Syphilis
- Chancroid
- Candidiasis
- Herpes simplex
- Scabies
- Lice
- Lymphogranuloma venereum
- Granuloma inguinale
- Molluscum contagiosum
- Trichomoniasis

Diseases notifiable throughout the UK except where specified: E, England; S, Scotland; W, Wales; NI, Northern Ireland

The Mental Health Act 1983

Section 2: ADMISSION FOR ASSESSMENT

Under section 2 of the Act, admission and detention of a patient for twenty-eight days may be made on the grounds that

a. he or she is suffering from mental disorder of a nature or degree which warrants the detention of the patient in a hospital for assessment (or for assessment followed by medical treatment) for at least a limited period and
b. he or she ought to be so detained in the interests of his or her own health or safety or with a view to the protection of other persons.

The application must be made by an approved social worker, or by the nearest relative, to the managers of the hospital to which admission is sought. The application must be supported by two registered medical practitioners, both of whom have examined the patient either together or within five days of each other. One medical recommendation must come from a practitioner who is approved by the Secretary of State as having special experience (as defined in section 12 of the Act). Both medical recommendations must support the grounds for admission (see above). A patient may be detained for a period not exceeding twenty-eight days. He then must be discharged or become an informal patient or a further compulsory detention order must be made. The patient may apply to a mental health review tribunal within fourteen days of admission (section 66).

Section 4: EMERGENCY ADMISSIONS

According to section 4 of the Act in any case of urgent necessity an application for admission for assessment for a period of up to seventy-two hours may be made either by an approved social worker or by the nearest relative of the patient. The applicant must state that it is of urgent necessity for the patient to be admitted and detained under section 2 (see above) and that compliance with the full provisions for compulsory detention would involve undesirable delay. One medical recommendation suffices given, if practicable, by a practitioner who has previous acquaintance with the patient. The certifying practitioner must have personally seen the patient within the previous twenty-four hours. The detention is valid for seventy-two hours but then expires unless a second medical recommendation (to comply with section 2) is given.

Section 135/136: PLACE OF SAFETY

An approved social worker (135) or a police officer (136) may remove anyone considered to be suffering from a mental disorder to 'a place of safety'. This may be a police station or a hospital. Further action can be taken under section 2, if required.

Abbreviated Mental Test Score

Each question scores one point

1. Age
2. Time (to nearest hour)
3. Address for recall at end of test (this should be repeated by patient to ensure it has been heard correctly)
4. Year
5. Name of hospital
6. Recognition of two persons (e.g. doctor, nurse)
7. Date of birth
8. Year of First World War
9. Name of present monarch
10. Count backwards 20 to 1

Lesions of peripheral nerves

AXILLARY (Circumflex) NERVE C5,6

Motor – Weakness or deltoid
Sensory – Anaesthesia of 'Regimental Badge' area of shoulder

RADIAL NERVE C5,6,7,8,T1

Injury in the axilla

Motor – Inability to extend elbow, wrist or fingers (if the hand is supported, the fingers can be extended by lubricals and interossei)
Wrist drop
Loss of triceps jerk
Sensory – Anaesthesia dorsum of forearm and patch over base of thumb

Injury in radial groove

Motor – As above except triceps is spared allowing elbow extension
Sensory – Anaesthesia of patch over base of thumb

MEDIAN NERVE C(5),6,7,8,T1

Injury at the elbow

Motor – Ulnar deviation when wrist is flexed against resistance
The index finger cannot be flexed at phalangeal joints (Pointing Sign)
Flexion of thumb at the interphalangeal joint is impossible
Thenar eminence muscle weakness

Sensory – Loss of sensation over palmar aspect of thumb and radial two fingers

Injury at wrist

Motor – Thenar eminence muscle weakness
Loss of abduction and opposition of thumb
Sensory – As above

ULNAR NERVE C8, T1

Injury at elbow

Motor – Weakness of flexor digitorum profundus – results in hyperextension of little and ring fingers at metacarpophalangeal joints
Paralysis of intrinsic muscles of hand (except thenar muscles and lateral two lumbricals) leading to inability to abduct and adduct fingers
Loss of adduction of thumb
Sensory – Loss of sensation over medial one and a half fingers – dorsum and palm

Injury at wrist

Motor – As above, but action of flexor digitorum profundus results in flexion of the interphalangeal joints and 'ulnar claw hand'
Sensory – Anaesthesia on palmar aspect of medial one and a half fingers

SCIATIC NERVE L4,5,S1,2,3

Motor – Loss of hamstring function
Complete paralysis below the knee (pull of gravity causes foot drop)
Loss of ankle jerk

Sensory – Complete loss below the knee except medial side of leg to big toe

COMMON PERONEAL NERVE L4,5,S1,2

Motor – Paralysis of extensor and peroneal groups leading to loss of dorsiflexion and eversion, foot drop

Sensory – Anaesthesia over anterior and lateral half of leg and dorsum of foot

FEMORAL NERVE L2,3,4

Motor – Weakness of quadriceps
Limited knee extension
Depressed knee jerk

Sensory – Anaesthesia over anterior thigh and medial aspect of leg

Assessment of motor power – MRC grading

0 = No active contraction can be detected
1 = Flicker of muscle contraction can be seen or felt by palpation over muscle, but activity insufficient to cause any joint movement
2 = Contraction is very weak but can just produce movement so long as weight of part can be countered by careful positioning of limb
3 = Contraction is still weak but can produce movement against gravitational resistance, e.g. quadriceps being able to extend knee with patient sitting
4 = Strength is not full but can produce movement against gravity and added resistance
5 = Normal power is present (compare one side with the other)

Reporting deaths to the Coroner

The doctor is advised to inform the Coroner about a death if:

- It cannot readily be certified as being due to natural causes
- The deceased was not seen by a doctor within the 14 days prior to death
- There is any element of suspicious circumstances
- There is any history of violence
- The death may be linked to an accident (whenever it occurred)
- There is any question of self-neglect or neglect by others
- The death has occurred or the illness arisen during or shortly after detention in police or prison custody (including voluntary attendance at a police station)
- The deceased was detained under the Mental Health Act
- The death is linked to an abortion
- The death might have been contributed to by the actions of the deceased himself (such as a history of drug or solvent abuse, self-injury or overdose)
- The deceased was receiving any form of war pension or industrial disability pension unless the death can be shown to be wholly unconnected
- The death could be due to industrial disease or related in any way to the deceased's employment
- The death was during an operation or before full recovery from the effects of the anaesthetic or was in any way related to the anaesthetic (in any event a death within 24 hours should normally be referred)
- The death may be related to a medical procedure or treatment whether invasive or not
- The death may be due to lack of medical care
- There are any other unusual or disturbing features to the case
- The death occurs within 24 hours of admission (unless the admission was purely for terminal care)
- It may be wise to report any death where there is an allegation of medical mismanagement

Trauma

Triage revised trauma score

		SCORE
RESPIRATORY (breaths/min)	10–29	**4**
	>29	**3**
	6–9	**2**
	1–5	**1**
	0	**0**
SYSTOLIC BP (mmHg)	>89	**4**
	76–89	**3**
	50–75	**2**
	1–49	**1**
	0	**0**
GLASGOW COMA SCALE	13–15	**4**
	9–12	**3**
	6–8	**2**
	4–5	**1**
	0	**0**

Glasgow Coma Scale (adults)

EYE OPENING

	POINTS
Spontaneous	**4**
To speech	**3**
To pain	**2**
Nil	**1**

BEST MOTOR RESPONSE

Obeys commands	**6**
Localizes to pain	**5**
Withdraws to pain	**4**
Abnormal flexor	**3**
Extensor response	**2**
Nil	**1**

VERBAL RESPONSE

Orientated	**5**
Confused conversation	**4**
Inappropriate words	**3**
Incomprehensible sounds	**2**
Nil	**1**

MAXIMUM POSSIBLE SCORE = 15
MINIMUM POSSIBLE SCORE = 3

Modified Glasgow Coma Scale in infants

EYE OPENING

	POINTS
Spontaneous	**4**
To speech	**3**
To pain	**2**
Nil	**1**

BEST MOTOR RESPONSE

Obeys commands	**6**
Localizes to pain	**5**
Withdraws to pain	**4**
Abnormal response	**3**
Extensor response	**2**
Nil	**1**

VERBAL RESPONSE

Appropriate words or social smiles, fixes on and follows objects	**5**
Cries but is consolable	**4**
Persistently irritable	**3**
Restless, agitated	**2**
Silent	**1**

Head injuries

INDICATIONS FOR SKULL X-RAY

1. Loss of consciousness or amnesia at any time
2. Neurological symptoms or signs
3. CSF from nose or ears
4. Suspected penetrating injury
5. Difficulty in assessing, e.g. young, epileptic or alcohol
6. Pronounced scalp bruising or swelling
7. Significant history

NOTE: Simple scalp laceration is not a criterion for X-ray.

INDICATIONS FOR ADMISSION TO HOSPITAL

1. Confusion or depression of level of consciousness at time of examination
2. Skull fracture
3. Neurological symptoms or signs
4. Difficulty assessing patient, e.g. young, epileptic or alcohol
5. Prolonged period of unconsciousness, e.g. 5 minutes
6. Other medical conditions, e.g. haemophilia
7. Lack of responsible adult to supervise

NOTE: Post-traumatic amnesia with full recovery is not an indication for admission.

INDICATIONS FOR CT SCAN NEUROSURGICAL OPINION

1. Fractured skull with confusion/altered state of consciousness, fits or neurological signs or symptoms
2. Coma persisting after resuscitation
3. Deterioration in level of consciousness
4. Confusion/neurological disturbance persistent over 8 hours even if no fracture visible
5. Compound depressed fracture or vault

6. Suspected fracture of base of skull
   - CSF leak
   - Orbital haematoma
   - Retromastoid haematoma
7. Penetrating injury

Burns: estimation of burn size

Lund and Browder chart
Ignore simple erythema

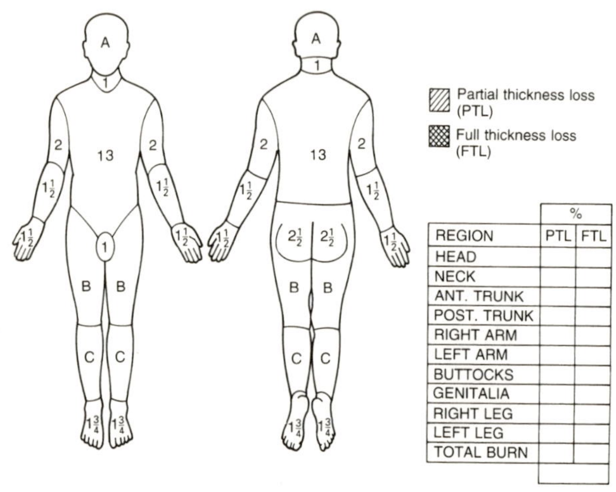

	%	
REGION	PTL	FTL
HEAD		
NECK		
ANT. TRUNK		
POST. TRUNK		
RIGHT ARM		
LEFT ARM		
BUTTOCKS		
GENITALIA		
RIGHT LEG		
LEFT LEG		
TOTAL BURN		

RELATIVE PERCENTAGE OF BODY SURFACE AREA AFFECTED BY GROWTH:

	Age (yr)					
Area	0	1	5	10	15	*Adult*
A = $\frac{1}{2}$ of HEAD	$9\frac{1}{2}$	$8\frac{1}{2}$	$6\frac{1}{2}$	$5\frac{1}{2}$	$4\frac{1}{2}$	$3\frac{1}{2}$
B = $\frac{1}{2}$ of THIGH	$2\frac{3}{4}$	$3\frac{1}{4}$	4	$4\frac{1}{2}$	$4\frac{1}{2}$	$4\frac{3}{4}$
C = $\frac{1}{2}$ of LEG	$2\frac{1}{2}$	$2\frac{1}{2}$	$2\frac{3}{4}$	3	$3\frac{1}{4}$	$3\frac{1}{2}$

Salter–Harris classification of epiphyseal fractures

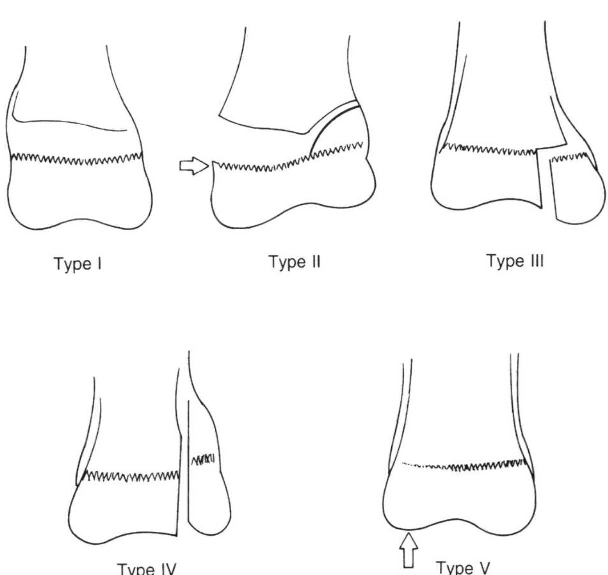

Sedation guidelines

DEFINITION

Technique in which the use of drug or drugs produces a state of depression of the CNS enabling treatment to be carried out, but during which communication is maintained such that the patient will respond to command throughout the period of sedation.

RECOMMENDATIONS

- The risk of each case should be assessed by the doctor prior to the procedure.
- Sedation must be carried out in a room where there are resuscitation facilities.
- All patients undergoing sedation require oxygen-enriched air.
- Patients undergoing sedation should have a cannula placed in a vein throughout the procedure.
- Pulse oximetry should become standard.
- Benzodiazepines are the most commonly used class of drugs for i.v. sedation and using careful titration technique they provide a wide margin of safety. The preferred drug is the shorter-acting midazolam.
- The use of a combination of benzodiazepines and opiates is not recommended.
- Specific antagonists for benzodiazepines (flumazenil) and opioids (naloxone) must be available for immediate use.
- There should be at least one other appropriately trained person (medical, nursing or technical) present.
- Monitoring should continue until recovery is complete.
- Minimum criteria for discharge include – ability to walk without support, stable vital signs, toleration of oral fluids, adequate analgesia and appropriate after-care.

Tetanus immunization

Immunization status	*Type of wound*	
	Clean	*Tetanus prone*
Last of 3 dose course, or reinforcing dose within last 10 years	Nil	Nil (A dose of adsorbed vaccine may be given if risk of infection is considered especially high)
Last of 3 dose course, or reinforcing dose more than 10 years previously	A reinforcing dose of adsorbed vaccine	A reinforcing dose of adsorbed vaccine plus a dose of human tetanus immunoglobulin
Not immunized or immunization status not known with certainty	A full 3 dose course of adsorbed vaccine	A full 3 dose course of vaccine, plus a dose of tetanus immunoglobulin

THE FOLLOWING ARE CONSIDERED TETANUS PRONE WOUNDS:

- Any wound or burns sustained more than 6 hours before surgical treatment.
- Any wound or burn at any interval after injury that shows one or more of the following characteristics:

  (i) A significant degree of devitalized tissue.
  (ii) Puncture type wound.
  (iii) Contact with soil or manure likely to harbour tetanus organisms.
  (iv) Clinical evidence of sepsis.

Thorough surgical toilet of the wound is essential whatever the tetanus immunization history of the patient.

CONTRAINDICATIONS

- Tetanus vaccine should not be given to an individual suffering from acute febrile illness except in the presence of a tetanus-prone wound. Minor infections without fever or systemic upset are not reasons to postpone immunization.
- Immunization should not proceed in individuals who have had a severe reaction to a previous dose.

Normal Values

Haematology

Haemoglobin	g/dl	Male	**13.5–18.0**
		Female	**11.5–16.5**
		Neonate	**17.0–22.0**
		Infant	**11.0–12.5**
		Child	**12.0–14.0**
		Pregnancy	**11.0–15.0**
Haematocrit (packed cell volume)		Male	**0.4–0.5**
		Female	**0.37–0.47**
		Child	**0.32–0.42**
Mean corpuscular volume	fl		**80–90**
Mean corpuscular Hb concentrate	g/dl		**30–40**
White cell count	$(\times 10^9/l)$	Adult	**4–11**
		Child	**5–15**
		Infant	**6–18**
		Neonate	**10–20**
Neutrophils	(% of WBC)		**50–70**
Lymphocytes	(% of WBC)		**20–45**
Platelets	$(\times 10^9/l)$		**150–400**
Bleeding time	minutes		**< 7**
Clotting time	minutes		**< 10**
Prothrombin time	seconds		**12–16**
Activated partial thromboplastin time	seconds		**32–36**

Biochemistry

		Serum values
Sodium (Na)		**137–150 mmol/l**
Potassium (K)		**3.5–5.5 mmol/l**
Chloride (Cl)		**97–108 mmol/l**
Urea		**3.5–7.5 mmol/l**
	Neonate	**1.7–5.3 mmol/l**
Creatinine		**60–100 μmol/l**
Bilirubin		**< 7 μmol/l**
Creatine (phospho) kinase		**< 200 i.u./l**
Amylase		**20–120 i.u./l**
Calcium		**2.2–2.7 mmol/l**
Protein total		**60–80 g/l**
Albumin		**35–55 g/l**
Globulin		**20–35 g/l**
Glucose (fasting)		**3.6–6.0 mmol/l**

Blood gases (arterial)

Oxygen	**10–13 kPa**	**(75–100 mmHg)**
Carbon dioxide	**4.6–6.0 kPa**	**(25–30 mmHg)**
pH	**7.36–7.44**	
H+ conc.	**36–44 nmol/l**	
Bicarbonate	**22–31 mmol/l**	
Base excess	**+/−2**	
Oxygen saturation	**0.96–1.00**	
Carboxyhaemoglobin (venous)	**< 6% saturation**	
NB: TOXIC	**> 20% saturation**	

Electrocardiogram

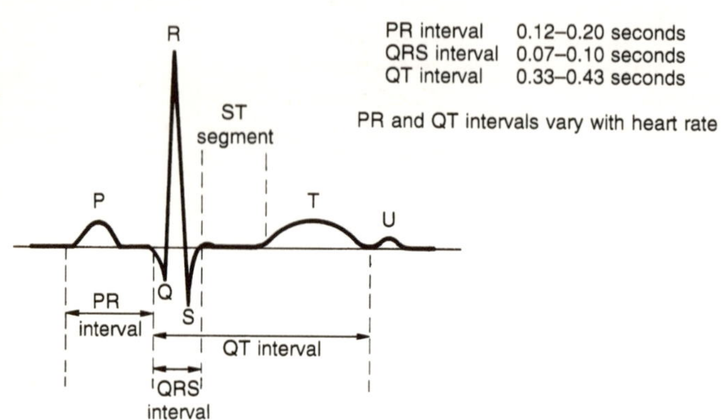

STANDARD ECG PAPER SPEED 25 mm/s
(5 large squares/s)
5 SMALL SQUARES = 0.2 s

P	Atrial depolarization
QRS	Ventricular depolarization
T	Ventricular repolarization
U	Slow repolarization of papillary muscles – inconstant feature

	Average	*Range*	
PR interval	0.18	0.12–0.20 s	beginning of P to beginning of QRS
QRS duration	0.08	up to 0.10 s	
QT interval	0.40	up to 0.42 s	
ST interval (QT – QRS)	0.32		

Approximate distribution of dermatomes

ANTERIOR ASPECT OF THE UPPER LIMB

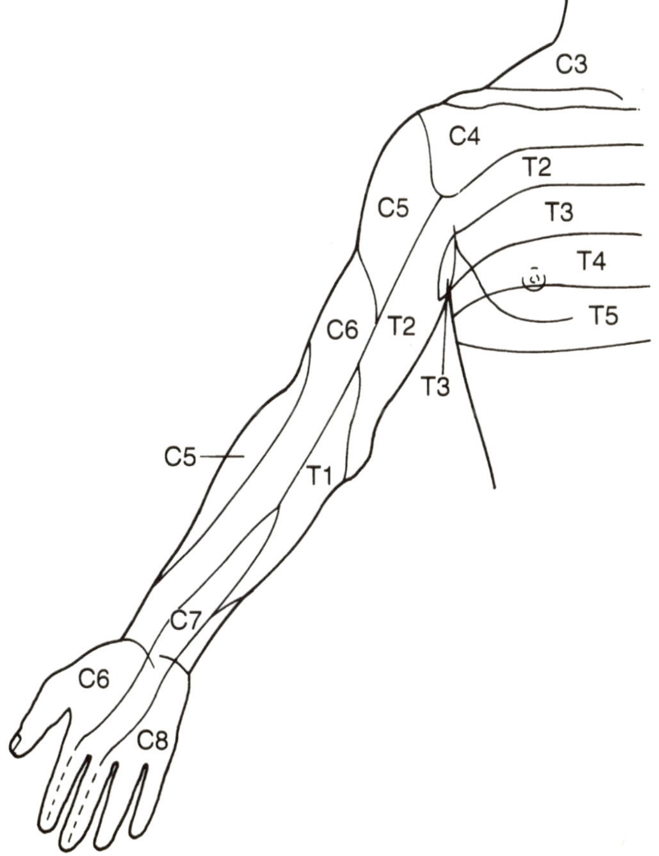

POSTERIOR ASPECT OF THE UPPER LIMB

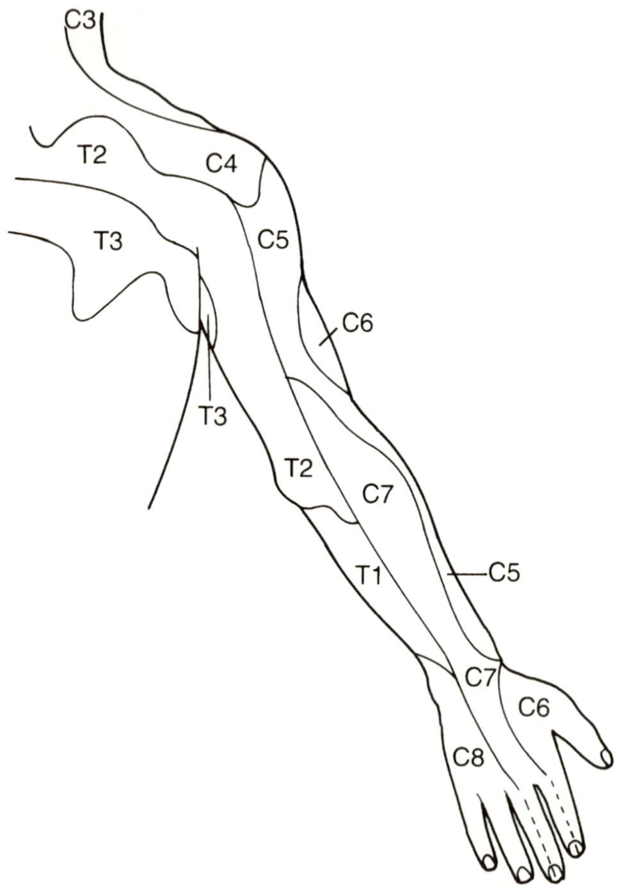

THE LOWER LIMB

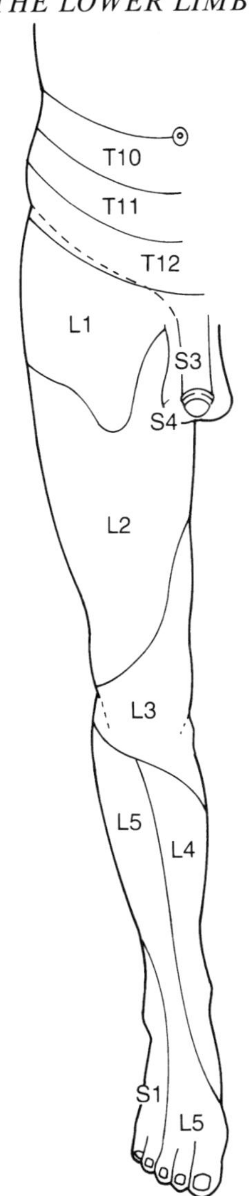

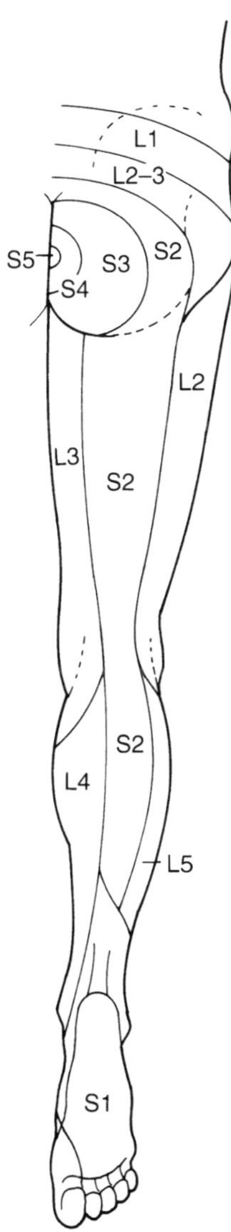

Pregnancy

UTERINE SIZE (FUNDAL HEIGHT)

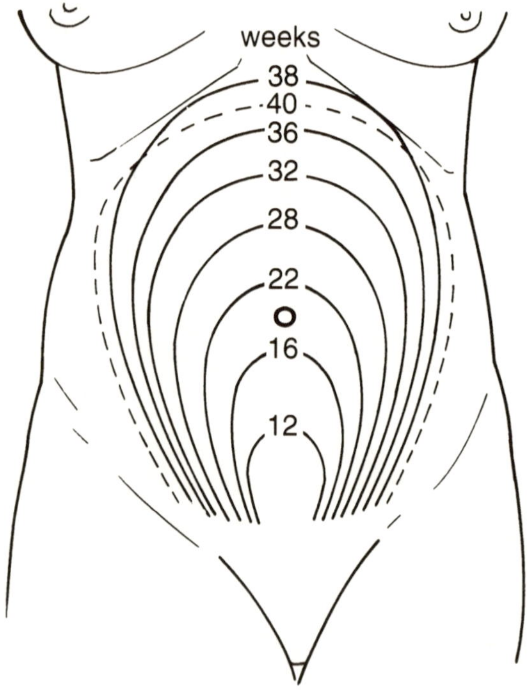

NB: 38–40 weeks reduction in fundal height due to descent of fetal head into pelvis.

QUICKENING

First fetal movements

- Primigravid 18 weeks
- Multipara 16–17 weeks

AUSCULTATION OF FETAL HEART WITH FETAL STETHOSCOPE

20 weeks: rate 120–160/minute.
(Doppler flowmeter can detect fetal heart sounds at 10–12 weeks.)

ESTIMATED DATE OF DELIVERY

1st day of last normal menstrual period + 9 months + 7 days.

PREGNANCY TESTS

Immunological Based on urinary beta-HCG excretion. Positive 8–9 days after first missed period.
Beta-HCG radioimmunoassay Detectable in serum 8–9 days after conception.
Ultrasound Can detect gestational sac at 5–6 weeks after last normal menstrual period.

Accessory ossicles in the foot

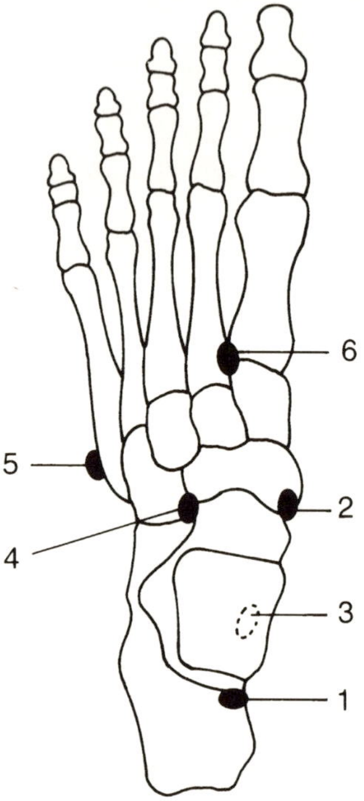

1. Os trigonum – 5%
2. Os tibiale (accessory navicular) – 10%
3. Os sustentaculi
4. Os calcaneus secundus
5. Os vesalium – 1%
6. Os cuneometatarseum
7. Os subtibiale (not shown – under medial malleolus) – 4%
8. Os subfibulare (not shown – under lateral malleolus) – 4%

There are other accessory ossicles that occur less frequently than the above.

Elbow development

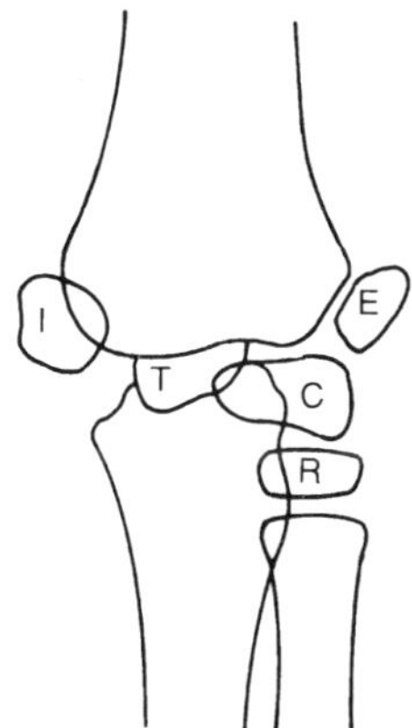

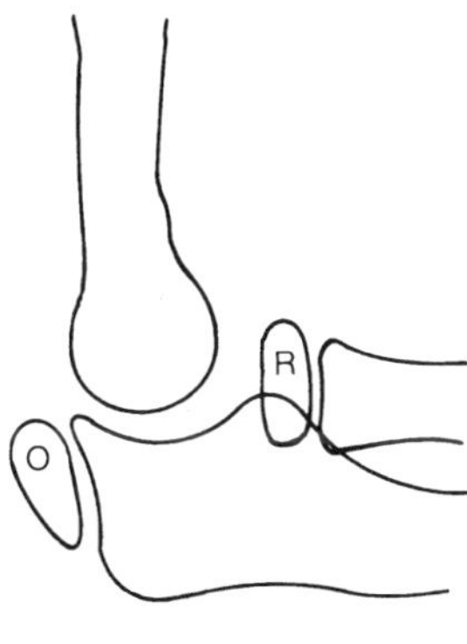

AVERAGE AGES OF APPEARANCE OF SECONDARY OSSIFICATION CENTRES

	Male	*Female*
C Capitellum	5 months	4 months
R Radial head	5 years	4 years
I Int. (medial) epicondyle	7 years	5 years
T Trochlea	9 years	8 years
O Olecranon	10 years	8 years
E Ext. (lateral) epicondyle	12 years	11 years

AVERAGE AGE OF FUSION

			Male	*Female*
Fusion of	C T E	to humeral shaft	17 yr	14 yr
	O	to ulna	18 yr	15 yr
	R	to radial shaft	15–17 yr	14–15 yr

Weight conversions

Stones	*Pounds*	*Kg*
0	7	3.2
1	0	6.4
1	7	9.6
2	0	12.8
2	7	16.0
3	0	19.2
3	7	22.4
4	0	25.6
4	7	28.8
5	0	32.0
5	7	35.2
6	0	38.4
6	7	41.6
7	0	44.8
7	7	48.0
8	0	51.2
8	7	54.4
9	0	57.6
9	7	60.8
10	0	64.0
10	7	67.2
11	0	70.4
11	7	73.6
12	0	76.8
12	7	80.0
13	0	83.2
13	7	86.4
14	0	89.6
14	7	92.8
15	0	96.0

Kilograms to pounds – multiply by 2.2

PAEDIATRIC WEIGHT ESTIMATES

4–8 years	$6 \times \text{age} + 12 = $ weight in pounds
8–12 years	$7 \times \text{age} + 5 = $ weight in pounds

Pharmacopoeia

Drugs A–Z

The following list of drugs is not intended to be a comprehensive pharmacopoeia. Further information should be obtained from the British National Formulary or from the manufacturer's data sheets. The infusion details are only suggestions and these may be adapted to local policies which in turn may be dependent on the equipment of delivery available in individual departments.

Drug	*Presentation*	*Notes*
Acetylcysteine *Paracetamol overdose* See Appendix		
i.v. infusion 150 mg/kg in 200 ml 5% glucose over 15 min then 50 mg/kg in 500 ml 5% glucose over 4 h then 100 mg/kg in 1000 ml 5% glucose over 16 h	Ampule 200 mg/ml 10 ml = 2 g/ampule	S/E: rashes, anaphylaxis
Adenosine *Supraventricular tachycardia* *Diagnosis of broad or narrow complex SVT*		
3 mg rapid i.v. injection over 2 seconds repeat with 6 mg then 12 mg if required after 1-2 minutes	Ampule 3 mg/ml 2 ml = 6 mg/ampule	NB: Patient on ECG monitor S/E: strange feelings, transient chest pain, bradycardia May cause bronchospasm, ECG rhythm disturbance Contraindication: asthma, 2nd- and 3rd-degree heart block, sick sinus syndrome interaction with dipyridamole
Adrenaline *Cardiac arrest*, see arrest protocol p. 3–5		
Anaphylaxis 0.5–1 mg i.m. injection of 1 in 1000 repeat 10 min intervals according to pulse and BP	Ampule 1 mg/ml 0.5 ml = 0.5 mg/Ampule 1 ml = 1 mg/Ampule	

Children less than	1 yr	0.05 ml i.m. (1 ml ampule diluted in 10ml N/saline give 0.5ml)
	1 yr	0.1 ml i.m.
	2 yr	0.2 ml i.m.
	3–4 yr	0.3 ml i.m.
	5 yr	0.4 ml i.m.
	6–12 yr	0.5 ml i.m.

Aminophylline
Reversible airway obstruction
Acute severe asthma

Slow i.v. injection (20 min)
250–500 mg (5 mg/kg)

Maintainance infusion 500 microgram/kg/h

Ampule 25 mg/ml
10 ml = 250 mg/ampule

S/E: tachycardia, arrhythmias, convulsions

NB: if on oral preparations convulsions and arrhythmias can occur before other signs of toxicity

70 kg patient
1 ampule (250 mg) in 500 ml of 5% glucose or N/saline = 0.5 mg/ml
500 microgram/kg/h = 35 ml/h

children slow i.v. injection (20 min) 5 mg/kg

Maintenance 6 month – 9 yr 1 mg/kg/h
10–16 yr 800 microgram/kg/h

Drug	Presentation	Notes
Amiodarone *Arrhythmia*		
Loading dose 5 mg/kg in 500 ml 5% glucose Not N/saline via central line over 20–120 minute Max 1.2 g in 24 h	Ampule 50 mg/ml 3 ml = 150 mg/ampule	NB: latent period before onset of action S/E: bradycardia, conduction disturbances, bronchospasm or apnoea in respiratory failure Avoid: in severe respiratory failure, CCF and severe arterial hypotension, pregnancy, breast feeding and sinus bradycardia
Amoxicillin *Community pneumonia*		
250 mg t.d.s. doubled in severe infection		NB: Penicillin sensitivity, rashes
Children up to 10 yr 125 mg t.d.s.		
i.v. injection 500 mg 8-hourly Children 50–100 mg/kg daily in divided doses		
Aspirin *Myocardial infarction*		
150 mg chewed		Contraindication: active GI bleeding, known aspirin sensitivity, anticoagulation
Atenolol *i.v. post myocardial infarction within 12 h*		
Slow i.v. injection 5–10 mg then 50 mg orally after 15 min 50 mg orally after 12 h then 100 mg daily	Ampule 500 microgram/ml 10 ml = 5 mg/ampule	S/E: bradycardia heart failure, bronchospasm, peripheral vasoconstriction Contraindication: obstructive airways disease, asthma, cardiogenic shock, sick sinus syndrome, 2nd- and 3rd-degree block

Arrhythmia		
2.5 mg i.v. at 1 mg/min repeated at 5 minute intervals to 10 mg max as required		
Atropine *Cardiac arrest* see p. 4		
Symptomatic bradycardia		
0.5–1 mg i.v.	Ampule 600 microgram/ml = 600 microgram/ ampule 100 microgram/ml 5 ml Min-I-Jet = 500 microgram	
Benzylpenicillin *Pneumonia*		
Slow i.v. injection 1.2 g daily in 4 divided doses Children 10–20 mg/kg daily in 4 divided doses 1 month – 12 years	Powder for reconstitution 600 mg ampule	NB: penicillin sensitivity
Meningitis		
Slow i.v. injection 2.4 g daily in 4 divided doses		
Children 1 month – 12 years 180–300 mg/kg daily in	4–6 divided doses	

Drug	Presentation	Notes
Bretylium *Cardiac arrest*, see p. 5		
Initial dose i.v. injection 5 mg/kg if successful (NB: up to 30 mins to take effect) then infusion 1–2 mg/min	Ampule 50 mg/ml 10 ml = 500 mg/ampule 10 ml Min-I-Jet = 50 mg/ml 500 mg	NB: may take up to 30 min to take effect, CPR must be continued for this period
	70 kg patient 1 ampule (500 mg) in 250 ml 5% glucose or N/saline = 2 mg/ml 1 mg/min = 30 ml/h	
Bupivacaine *Local anaesthetic*, see p. 100		
Calcium *Cardiac arrest*, see p. 5		
10 ml 10% calcium chloride	Min-I-Jet 100 mg/ml 10 ml = 1 g/syringe	
20–30 ml 10% calcium gluconate	Ampule 5 ml, 10 ml	

Drug / indication / dose	Preparation	Notes
Cefotaxime *Compound fracture* 1 g t.d.s. 2 g t.d.s. in severe infection	Powder for reconstitution 500 mg ampule	
Children 100–150 mg/kg daily in 2–4 divided doses In severe infections up to 100 mg/kg daily		
Charcoal *Poisoning* Carbomix 50 g adult 25 g children (50 g in severe poisoning)		
Medicoal effervescent (5 g sachet) 1–2 sachet repeated every 15–20 min until charcoal given is 5–10 times poison dose if known or 50 g		
Chlorpheniramine *Anaphylaxis*		
s.c. or i.m. injection 10–20 mg repeated if required max. 40 mg/24 h	Ampule 10 mg/ml 1 ml = 10 mg/ampule	S/E: injection may be irritant, transient hypotension or CNS stimulation
Slow i.v. injection over 1 min 10–20 mg diluted in syringe with 5–10 ml of patient's blood (or N/Saline or water for injection – both unlicensed dilutents)		

Drug	*Presentation*	*Notes*
Chlorpromazine *Quietens disturbed patients whatever underlying psychopathology*		
Deep i.m. injection 25–50 mg	Ampule 25 mg/ml 1 ml = 25 mg/ampule 2 ml = 50 mg/ampule	S/E: large number of side-effects of note: hypotension, ECG changes, tachycardia and arrhythmias NB: exclude hypoxia, hypotension as cause of agitation Avoid skin contact –sensitization reported
Co-amoxiclav *Soft tissue infection*		
Dose expressed as amoxicillin		
250 t.d.s., doubled in severe infections Children under 6 yr 5 ml of 125 mg suspension t.d.s. 6–12 yr 5 ml of 250 mg suspension t.d.s.		
i.v. injection 1 g t.d.s. Children 3 months – 12 years 25 mg/kg t.d.s.	Powder for reconstitution 600 mg (500 mg amoxicillin) 1.2 g (1 g amoxicillin)	NB: penicillin sensitivity Caution in pregnancy, breast feeding, hepatitis, hepatic impairment.
Cyclizine *Anti-emetic with slow i.v. injection*		
Adult 50 mg Children 6–12 yr 25 mg	Ampule 50 mg/ml 1 ml = 50 mg/ampule	S/E: drowsiness may aggravate severe heart failure

Diamorphine *Acute pain*		
s.c. or i.m. injection 5–10 mg Slow i.v. injection 2.5–5 mg	Powder for reconstitution	S/E: nausea, vomiting, hypotension, respiratory depression NB: specific antagonist **Naloxone**, see p. 103
Children slow i.v. injection 3–6 months 25–50 microgram/kg 6–12 months 75 microgram/kg over 12 months 75–100 microgram/kg		
Myocardial infarction		
Slow i.v. injection 5 mg then 2.5–5 mg if required (elderly and frail half dose)		
Acute pulmonary oedema		
Slow i.v. injection 2.5–5 mg		
Diazepam *Convulsions*		
Slow i.v. injection 10–20 mg at 1 mg/min children 0.25 mg/kg at 1 mg/min	Ampule 5 mg/ml 2 ml = 10 mg/ampule	S/E: respiratory depression NB: beware low cardiac output states – very slow onset of action
p.r. 0.5 mg/kg	Rectal tube 2 mg/ml 2.5 ml = 5 mg/tube	NB: specific antagonist **flumazenil**, see p. 98
Sedation 5–10 mg i.v. titrated to effect	Rectal tube 4 mg/ml 2.5 ml = 10 mg/tube	

Drug	*Presentation*	*Notes*
Digoxin *Fast atrial fibrillation*		
0.75–1 mg i.v. in 50 ml 5% glucose or N/saline over 2 or more hours	Ampule 250 microgram/ml 2 ml = 500 microgram/ampule	S/E: nausea, arrhythmias NB: beware of hypokalaemia
Disopyramide *Ventricular arrhythmias especially after MI and SVT*		Contraindication: heart block 2nd/3rd, severe heart failure
Slow i.v. injection 2 mg/kg over at least 5 min to maximum of 150 mg followed immediately by 200 mg orally then 200 mg orally every 8 h for 24 h	Ampule 10 mg/ml 5 ml = 50 mg/ampule	S/E: myocardial depression, hypotension, AV block NB: ECG monitoring
OR 400 microgram/kg/h i.v. to a maximum of 300 mg in the first hour and 800 mg daily	Capsules 100 mg/150 mg	

70 kg patient
5 ampules (250 mg) in 250 ml of 5% glucose or N/saline = 1 mg/ml
70kg × 0.4 = 28mg/ml
400 microgram/kg/h = 28 ml/h

Dobutamine
Cardiogenic shock

2.5–10 microgram/kg/min Titrate dose to response	Ampule 12.5 mg/ml 20 ml = 250 mg/ampule	S/E: risk exists of increasing oxygen demand of myocardium beyond supply, Tachycardia and marked increase in systotic blood pressure indicate overdosage.

70 kg patient
1 ampule (250 mg) in 250 ml of 5% glucose or N/saline = 1 mg/ml
5 microgram/kg/min = 350 microgram/min = 0.35 ml/min = 21 ml/h

Dopamine
Cardiogenic shock
Renal protection

Ionotropic dose 3–10 microgram/kg/min Renal dose 1–3 microgram/kg/min	Ampule 40 mg/ml 5 ml = 200 mg/ampule	S/E: risk of myocardial oxygen demand increasing beyond demand Peripheral vasoconstriction
Titrate dose to response	or 160 mg/ml 5 ml = 800 mg/ampule	

70 kg patient
1 × 200 mg ampule (200mg) in 200 ml of 5% glucose or N/saline = 1mg/ml
3 microgram/kg/min = 210 microgram/min = 0.21 ml/min = 12.6ml/h

Drug	*Presentation*	*Notes*
Erythromycin *Alternative to penicillin in hypersensitive patients* *Atypical pneumonias*		
Adult and child over 8 years 250 mg q.d.s. Children up to 2 years 125 mg q.d.s. 2–8 years 250 mg q.d.s. Doses doubled in severe infections	Powder for reconstitution 1 g ampule	S/E: nausea
i.v. infusion adult and child severe infections 50 mg/kg daily by continuous infusion or divided doses every 6 h		
Flecainide *Resistant ventricular tachycardia* *Wolff–Parkinson–White accessory pathway arrhythmia* *Disabling atrial fibrillation*		
Slow i.v. injection over 10–30 min 2 mg/kg to a maximum of 150 mg followed by infusion if necessary 1.5 mg/kg/h for 1h then reducing to 100–250 microgram/kg/h for up to 24 h Maximum cumulative dose in first 24 h 600 mg	Ampule 10 mg/ml 15 ml = 150 mg/ampule	Caution: pacemakers avoid in condition defect atrial, 2nd degree or greater AV block, bundle branch block Contraindication: heart failure, myocardial infarction S/E: dizziness, arrhythmias

70 kg patient
50 ml (500 mg) in 500 ml of 5% glucose or N/saline
= 1 mg/ml
100 ml over first hour then 10–25 ml/h if required

Flucloxacillin *Soft tissue infections*		
250 mg q.d.s. orally Slow i.v. injection 0.25–1 g every 6 h Double dose in severe infection	Powder for reconstitution	NB: penicillin sensitivity
Children any route under 2 years quarter adult dose 2–10 years half adult dose		

Drug	Presentation	Notes
Flumazenil *Reversal of sedative effect of benzodiazepines (Not licensed in self overdose)*		
i.v. injection of 200 microgram over 15 s Then 100 microgram at 60 s intervals if required Usual dose range 300–600 microgram Maximum total is 1 mg (2 mg on ITU)	Ampule 100 μg/ml 5 ml = 500 μg/ampule	NB: short-acting – repeated doses may be necessary. Too rapid reversal can cause agitation and fear. Question aetiology if there is no response to repeated doses
Glucagon *Acute hypoglycaemia*		
s.c. or i.m. or i.v. injection Used in adults and children 0.5–1 unit (1 unit = 1 mg glucagon)	Powder for reconstitution 1 unit ampule or 10 unit ampule	NB: if no response after 15 minutes i.v. glucose should be given
Hydrocortisone *hypersensitivity reaction,* *asthma (if not able to take oral prednisolone)*		
i.m. or slow i.v. injection 100-200 mg	Powder for reconstitution – 100 mg	
Ipecacuanha *Induction of emesis in selected patients* Adult 30 ml Child 6–18 months 10 ml with water over 18 months 15 ml with water Repeat after 20 min if necessary		S/E: vomiting can be excessive Caution: avoid in ingestion of corrosive or petroleum products

Ipratropium bromide
Reversible airways obstruction

Inhalation of nebulized solution 100–500 microgram (0.4–2 ml of a 0.025% solution)	Ampule 0.025% = 250 microgram/ml 2ml = 500 microgram	Caution: in glaucoma If further dilution is required use sterile N/saline

Isoprenaline
Symptomatic bradycardia unresponsive to atropine

0.5–10 microgram/min i.v. infusion	Ampule 1 mg/ml 2 ml = 2 mg/ampule 20 microgram/ml Min-I-Jet 10 ml = 200 microgram/syringe	S/E: tachycardia, hypotension, arrhythmias

Infusion
2.5 ampules, 5 ml (5 mg) in 500 ml of 5% glucose or N/saline
= 10 microgram/ml
5 microgram/min = 0.5 ml/min = 30 ml/h

Drug	Presentation	Notes
Lignocaine *Local anaesthetic*, see below		
Ventricular tachycardia		
100 mg (in patient without gross myocardial depression) as bolus over few minutes Followed by infusion 2–4 mg/min	Ampule 1%, 2% Min-I-Jet 1% 10 ml = 100 mg/syringe Infusion 0.1% (1 mg/ml) 0.2% (2 mg/ml)	S/E: confusion, convulsions Caution: in congestive cardiac failure Contraindication: all grades of AV block, severe myocardial depression
LOCAL ANAESTHETICS		
Bupivacaine *Toxic dose* 2 mg/kg (plain) 3 mg/kg (with adrenaline)		Toxic effects of local anaesthetics are usually associated with excessive plasma levels. This is dependent upon route of administration and intravascular injection must be avoided at all times. Vasoconstrictor must not be used in digits and appendages.
Lignocaine *Toxic dose* 3 mg/kg (plain) 7 mg/kg (with adrenaline)		S/E: CNS excitation, convulsions, followed by depression. Cardiovascular depression and arrhythmia

Prilocaine
Toxic dose 6 mg/kg (plain) 8 mg/kg (with adrenaline)

1% = 1 g/100 ml
= 1000 mg/100 ml
= 10 mg/ml

Concentration (mg/ml) can be calculated from percentage value as above or by moving the decimal point of the percentage concentration one place to the right

e.g. 1% solution contains 10 mg/ml
2% solution contains 20 mg/ml

Mannitol
Osmotic diuresis for cerebral oedema

1 g/kg as a 20% solution given by rapid i.v. infusion	20% infusion 200 mg/ml 1g = 5ml	Caution: extravasation causes inflammation and thrombophlebitis Contraindication: congestive cardiac failure, pulmonary oedema

Drug	*Presentation*	*Notes*
Metoclopramide *Anti-emetic used with opiate analgesia*		
i.m. injection or i.v. injection over 1–2 min		
Adult 10 mg Children	Ampule 5 mg/ml 2 ml = 10 mg/ampule	S/E: extrapyramidal effects especially in children and young adults Daily dose must not exceed 500 microgram/kg

Age	*Weight*	*Dose*
0–3 yr	0–14 kg	1 mg
3–5 yr	15–19 kg	2 mg
5–9 yr	20–29 kg	2.5 mg
9–14 yr	30 kg +	5 mg

Drug	*Presentation*	*Notes*
Metronidazole *Anaerobic infection*		
Orally 800 mg initially then 400 mg every 8 h		
i.v. infusion 500 mg every 8 h	Infusion 5 mg/ml 100 ml bag = 500 mg/bag	Caution: disulfiram-like reaction with alcohol S/E: nausea and vomiting
Children (any route) 7.5 mg/kg every 8 h		

Midazolam *Sedation*		
2 mg i.v. injection over 30 s (1–1.5 mg in elderly) after 2 min can be followed by 0.5–1 mg increments Usual dosage range 2.5–7.5 mg (1–2 mg in the elderly)	Ampule 2 mg/ml 5 ml = 10 mg/ampule 5 mg/ml 2 ml = 10 mg/ampule	S/E: respiratory depression, hypotension Beware: low cardiac output states cause slow onset of action NB: specific antagonist **flumazenil**, see p. 98
Morphine *Acute pain*		
s.c. or i.m. injection 10 mg Children up to 1 month 150 microgram/kg 1–12 months 200 microgram/kg 1–5 years 2.5–5 mg 6–12 years 5–10 mg Slow (2 mg/min) i.v. injection quarter to half i.m. dose	Ampule 10, 15, 20, 30 mg/ml all 2 ml = 20, 30, 40 and 60 mg/ampule	S/E: respiratory depression, nausea NB: specific antagonist **naloxone**, see below
Naloxone *Specific opiate antagonist*		
Adult 0.8–2 mg i.v. repeated every 2–3 min to a maximum of 10 mg Children 10 microgram/kg with subsequent dose of 100 microgram/kg Can also be given s.c. or i.m.	Ampule 400 microgram/ml 1 ml = 400 microgram/ampule	NB: short duration of action repeated doses may be required. Question aetiology if no response to repeated doses

Drug	*Presentation*	*Notes*
Nitrates *Unstable angina* *Analgesia for acute myocardial infarction* *Left ventricular failure*		
Sublingua: 0.3–1 mg repeated as required Nitrolingual spray 400 metered dose Buccal tablets 3–5 mg. Remove if fall in blood pressure	Tablets 300 microgram/ 500 microgram	S/E: hypotension, headaches
Patches 5/10 mg i.v. infusion 10–200 microgram/min Glyceryl trinitrate Isosorbide dinitrate i.v. infusion 2–10 mg/h	Numerous preparations see specific data sheet	

Non-steroidal anti-inflammatory drugs (NSAIDs)
e.g. sodium diclofenac, ibuprofen

Numerous and variable, can be given by many routes, orally, topically, i.m., p.r.

Caution: in elderly, allergic disorders especially salicylate hypersensitivity, asthma. Avoid in pregnancy.
S/E: GI discomfort, occasionally bleeding and ulceration, angio-oedema, asthma and rashes

CSM advice (peptic ulceration)
NSAIDs should not be given to patients with acute peptic ulceration. In patients with a history of peptic ulceration and in the elderly they should be given only after other forms of treatment have been carefully considered.
In all patients it is prudent to start at the bottom end of the dosage range.

CSM advice (asthma)
Any degree of worsening of asthma may be related to the ingestion of NSAID, either prescribed or purchased over the counter.

Drug	*Presentation*	*Notes*
Paraldehyde *Status epilepticus*		
Deep i.m. injection. Single dose. Usual dose 5–10 ml, max 20 ml. NO more than 5 ml at any site.	Ampule 5 ml and 10 ml	Caution: Do not use if brown or with acetic acid odour. Avoid contact with rubber and plastic. S/E: rash, pain, sterile abscess, avoid sciatic nerve
Children: *Age* / *Dose* 0–3 mth 0.5 ml 3–6 mth 1 ml 6–12 mth 1.5 ml 1–2 yr 2 ml 3–5 yr 3–4 ml 6–12 yr 5–6 ml		rectal irritation after enema
Rectal: adult 5–10 ml as 10% enema in N/Saline Child as per i.m. dose		
Pethidine *Acute pain*		
Slow i.v. injection 25–50 mg repeated after 4 h s.c. i.m. injection 25–100 mg	50 mg/ml 1 ml = 50 mg/ampule	S/E: respiratory depression, nausea and vomiting NB: specific antagonist **naloxone**, see p. 103
Children 0.5–2 mg/kg		
Phenytoin *Digoxin-induced arrhythmias* *Third-line treatment in paediatric convulsions* *Status epilepticus in adults*		
Loading dose 10–15 mg/kg over 20–30 min with ECG and blood pressure monitoring For a 70 kg man this is 700 mg–1.05 g which is 3–4 ampoules	Ampule 50 mg/ml 5 ml amp. (250 mg)	S/E: cardiovascular, central nervous system and respiratory depression, arrhythmias, hypotension

Prilocaine
Local anaesthetic, see p. 101

Procyclidine
Acute dystonia and oculogyric crisis

i.m. 5–10 mg repeated after 20 min if necessary. Maximum 20 mg/day i.v. 5 mg usually effective within 5 min. Occasionally the patient may need 10 mg and up to 30 min for relief of symptoms	Ampules 5 mg/ml 2 ml amps (10 mg/amp.)	S/E: GI disturbance, urinary retention, tachycardia, mental confusion Contraindication: glaucoma (closed angle)

Salbutamol
Reversible airway obstruction

Inhalation of nebulized solution 2.5–5 mg (may be diluted with N/saline) Repeat up to 10 mg if side-effects permit Children 2.5 mg increasing to 5 mg if necessary	Ampule 1 mg/ml 2mg/ml 2.5 ml = 2.5 and 5 mg/ampule	S/E: tachycardia; peripheral vasodilatation Caution: in hypertensives, myocardial insufficiency, arrhythmias
Slow i.v. injection of 250 micrograms over 20 minutes. Repeated if necessary. i.v. infusion 5 microgram/min adjusting depending on effect and side effect. Usual range 3-20 microgram/min	Ampule 500 microgram/ml 1ml = 500 microgram/ampule Ampule 1mg/ml 1ml = 1mg/ampule 5ml = 5mg/ampule	

> Infusion
> 5 ampules (5 mg) in 500 ml of 5% glucose or N/saline = 10 microgram/ml
> 3–20 microgram/min = 0.3–2 ml/min = 18–120 ml/h

Drug	*Presentation*	*Notes*
Sodium bicarbonate *Severe metabolic acidosis*		
Adult pH less than 7.0 during or immediately following cardiac arrest		
$\frac{\text{Base excess} \times \text{weight (kg)}}{3} = \text{mmol } 8.4\%$	8.4% solution 1 mmol = 1 ml	Caution: avoid in respiratory acidosis
Children 1 mmol/kg		
Tetanus toxoid *Tetanus vaccination*		
see p. 67 Tetanus vaccine 0.5ml deep i.m. injection	Ampule 0.5 ml	Contraindication: Known allergy NB: Vaccination should be postponed if patient is acutely ill, minor infection without fever or systemic upset are not contraindications

Tetanus immunoglobulin
Treatment tetanus or tetanus prone wound

see p. 67
i.m. injection 250 units increasing to 500 units if greater than 24 h have elapsed or if there is risk of heavy contamination

Treatment of established tetanus is 150 units/kg in multiple injection sites

Verapamil
Supraventricular tachycardia

Slow i.v. injection 5–15 mg diluted to 1 mg/ml with N/saline A further 5 mg can be given 5–10 min later if required	Ampule 2.5 mg/ml 2 ml = 5 ml/ampule	NB: ECG-monitor Caution: Drug interaction with digoxin and beta blockers i.v. can cause asystole S/E: Headaches, flushing, hypotension

Appendix Preparation of acetylcysteine

1st infusion 200 ml 5% glucose over 15 min
2nd infusion 500 ml 5% glucose over 4 h
3rd infusion 1000 ml 5% glucose over 16 h

	ml (number of ampules) Parvolax		
Body weight (kg)	*1st*	*2nd*	*3rd*
40	30 (3.0)	10 (1.0)	20 (2.0)
44	33 (3.3)	11 (1.1)	22 (2.2)
48	36 (3.6)	12 (1.2)	24 (2.4)
52	39 (3.9)	13 (1.3)	26 (2.6)
56	42 (4.2)	14 (1.4)	28 (2.8)
60	45 (4.5)	15 (1.5)	30 (3.0)
64	48 (4.8)	16 (1.6)	32 (3.2)
68	51 (5.1)	17 (1.7)	34 (3.4)
72	54 (5.4)	18 (1.8)	36 (3.6)
76	57 (5.7)	19 (1.9)	38 (3.8)
80	60 (6.0)	20 (2.0)	40 (4.0)
84	63 (6.3)	21 (2.1)	42 (4.2)
88	66 (6.6)	22 (2.2)	44 (4.4)
90	69 (6.9)	23 (2.3)	46 (4.6)

Additional Data

Useful telephone numbers

Accident & Emergency: Dept . . . .
Office . . . .
Reception . . . .

Bacteriology . . . .
Biochemistry . . . .
Blood Bank . . . .
Coronary Care . . . .
Coroner's Office . . . .
Dining Room . . . .
Fracture Clinic . . . .
Haematology . . . .
Health Visitor . . . .
ITU . . . .
Medical Records . . . .
Medical Staffing/Personnel . . . .
Mortuary . . . .
Occupational Therapy . . . .
Out-Patients . . . .
Paediatric Liaison . . . .
Pharmacy . . . .
Physiotherapy . . . .
Social Services . . . .
Theatres . . . .
Toxicology . . . .
X-ray . . . .
Wards . . . .
. . . .
. . . .
. . . .
. . . .
. . . .

Others . . . .
. . . .
. . . .
. . . .
. . . .
. . . .

Local data/information

Index